An American Epidemic:

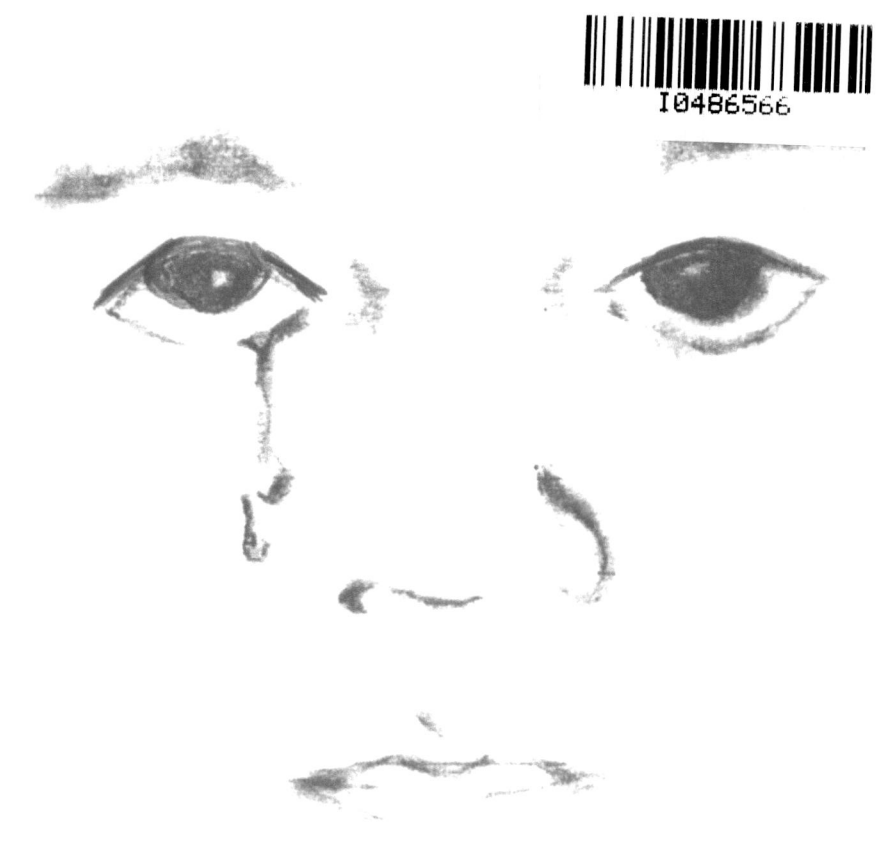

Lil' White Lies

Al Evans III
Cover Design by Cory Evans
Illustration by Steaven "Tae" Evans

Order this book online at www.trafford.com
or email orders@trafford.com

Most Trafford titles are also available at major online book retailers.

Portion of proceeds will go to:
CASA Coalition Against Sexual Abuse
"Mi casa es su casa. My house is your house"
Providing a safe haven for victims of child sexual abose

Casa is an organization of volunteers, survivors of child sexual assault, their
families and friends, and professionals dedicated to raise awareness about child
rape, molestation and incest, and to offer services for empowerment.

Print information available on the last page.

ISBN: 978-1-4120-4792-0 (sc)

Trafford rev. 01/17/2020

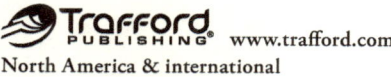
www.trafford.com
North America & international
toll-free: 1 888 232 4444 (USA & Canada)
fax: 812 355 4082

*This book is dedicated to
my Mother, Sarah Alice,
may she rest in peace*

and to all the Children of the world

———————————

The Purpose Of This Book

- Reveal the epidemic of child sexual abuse in Utah.
- Uncover the reasons behind this crisis.
- Suggest ways to:
  Empower and protect children
  Educate and heal adults
  Expose and punish perpetrators

NOTE: The names of the survivors of child sexual abuse in the accounts that follow have been changed to protect them and promote their potential for healing. Slander and libel laws prevent me from using the full names of perpetrators who have not been tried and convicted or, believe me, I would. Keep in mind, however, that the truth is always a defense against libel. These stories are true as told to me from the hearts and mouths of the survivors themselves.

Chapter 1

Maybe It Takes A Stranger

Mom was visiting my family and I back East when two weeks before she was to return to Utah, she asked me: "Three, Why don't you come to Utah? "

"Come to Utah?" I said. "Why would I want to go to Utah?"

"Just come to Utah," she said. At the time, I did not know my mother was dying of cancer.

I told her, "Well, give me a week to think about it."

So, for seven days I prayed, thought about it, prayed and thought about leaving home. Then the revelation hit me like 3 tons of bricks – Go! Go to Utah! I had one week to make arrangements. I sold my iguana and got rid of my furniture.

I went to the airport to get a ticket. I had too much baggage. I laughed along with the agent when she said, "You can't move across country by plane!" I had to figure out what I was going to do with all of my extras. Well, the plane was out. I would have to go by bus.

A day later, I took a Greyhound bus headed West with six pieces of luggage, 80 cents in my pocket and two hamburgers in a paper bag. I had no idea how long I would be gone.

I took the last bite of my last burger about 30 miles outside of Salt Lake City two and a half days later. As I walked outside the bus station, trying to hail a cab (I had no idea this was prohibited), the air was crisp, cold and clear. Bright blue skies. I stepped into the middle of the street waving at a cab on the other side, when I looked up and yelled, "Wow! Look at those mountains!" They stopped me in my tracks.

People passed by looking at me and laughing. It was obvious that I was not from around here.

Those giant rocks held up the eastern sky. They were dominant, unyielding, a thing of nature to be noticed. The Utah Rocky Mountains demanded my attention and awe. I didn't know then that in the next four years those mountains would become a symbol for what I grew to understand I must do here. Like them, I would have to be unyielding no matter the consequences of exposing Utah's dirty little secret, a sickness that slithers like a contaminated river from those majestic mountains.

I'm Not From Around Here

Before I came to Utah to care for my mother, I had never met a Mormon. But I learned in a very short time how every facet of Utah society is shaped by the beliefs and practices of the Church of Jesus Christ of Latter-day Saints (LDS church), whose members are commonly called Mormons.

Once a small Utah sect, Mormons now comprise a global church worth an estimated $25 billion with 11 million members worldwide, a slight majority of them living outside the United States. The 1990 census showed 1,236,242 Mormons in Utah made up 72% of the state's total 1.7 million population. The official population of Utah is now 2.3 million, according to 2000 census reports. Utah is growing the fourth fastest of all 50 states. The state grew 30% from 1990 to 2000, adding more than a half-million people, compared with the overall growth rate of 13% in the United States.

As in prior census years, Utah continues to have *the youngest population of all 50 states.* Nearly one-third of the population was under 18 years old in 2000. This reflects the strong emphasis the LDS church puts on its members having large families.

2

The church teaches Mormons not to smoke, use illicit drugs, drink alcohol or any beverages with caffeine, participate in premarital sex or masturbation, watch R-rated movies or cuss. Members should dress modestly and conservatively. They pride themselves in projecting a wholesome Christian image. Doctrine emphasizes marriage and family as the cornerstone of the church and society. The LDS church also has a highly organized welfare and work-support program financed in part by tithing donations made by members who pay 10% of their gross income to the church each month.

Mormonism began when 14-year-old Joseph Smith said God and Jesus Christ visited him in 1820 in upstate New York, telling him not to join any of the existing churches. Smith also said an angel named Moroni appeared to him in 1823 and revealed where he could dig up "the Golden Plates" from which he supposedly translated what is now known as *The Book of Mormon – Another Testament of Jesus Christ*. These "visions" led Smith to establish a new church in 1830 that would teach the "restored" gospel of Jesus Christ, claiming it as the "only true" church on Earth.

In my time here, I've been blessed to meet many warm, generous and genuinely caring people, Mormons and non-Mormons alike. However, it is evident to any person of color that Utah is an extremely racist and very strange place to be.

For a while I sang and played in a band here, and I wasn't really surprised when my guitarist asked me, "What would make a black person stay in Utah, considering how racist Utah is?" That's a good question. Diversity is not valued here, it is feared. Not only are people discriminated against because they are not white but, just as backwards and appalling, because they are not members of the dominant religion.

I listen to people. This is what I do. It's who I am. It's what I've done all my life. As a student of human nature, I've had the opportunity to work in mental health counseling and direct care the past 25 years. I watch and observe people, let them talk, and sometimes advise them to help them through their most difficult times. My instincts are usually correct.

My second week in Utah, I had this overwhelming feeling that something was not right about this place.

People seemed muted. Their joy plastic. Their pain masked. Many of those I talked with seemed emotionally anesthetized. Others were hostile toward or intimidated by independent thought and personal power. Anyone different from them with a strong sense of self was viewed with suspicion.

Maybe it takes a stranger, someone from the outside looking in, to see an evident flaw in a society as sheltered as that of Utah's majority population.

After my mother's death, I wanted to leave. I stayed because nearly every day I met someone who told me the same horrifying story. Person after person, all Utah natives, said they were molested or raped beginning at a young age mostly by male members of the LDS church but by women, too. The abusers were most often family or church members. Over the past four years, I have interviewed hundreds of victims here. In my lifetime, I've been around the world twice, studying cultures, talking with indigenous people to discover what makes them unique. In all my travels, across the United States and the globe, I have never once run into such a serious disease innate to a particular society as child sexual abuse is to Utah.

"Little" White Lies

Being African American in a country haunted by slavery and bigotry, I grew up hearing *black* and *dark* associated with all things negative and evil. Innocent people were *blackmailed* or *black-balled.* Or someone hid a *deep, dark secret.* Meanwhile, a *white* lie was considered small and not too damaging.

Utah's white lies, however, are not insignificant. These white lies feed the disease of child sexual abuse that preys on innocent victims who have no voice and no power.

This is a reality that the white-male dominated LDS church can no longer ignore. I emphasize "white-male" because there are no others – brown, yellow, red, black or female – in power in the Mormon church. The church's inability, refusal or incompetence in dealing with decades of child molestation, rape and incest within its congregation and society is a failure of colossal proportions. The fact this epidemic has gone on so long, and is allowed or tolerated, shows an internal weakness not only in the church's practices, teachings and beliefs but also in the state's culture, law enforcement and justice system.

4

Mormons may not want to claim this as their problem. After all, church authorities might say, LDS doctrine teaches sexual abstinence before marriage. Mormonism has stringent moral laws against masturbation, homosexuality and adolescent sexual petting or foreplay. People who molest their children must not be true members of the church.

Let's be clear. This is very much an LDS problem.

If you don't believe me, ask. Ask your friends and neighbors, your Sunday school teachers and church members, your old missionary companions, your siblings, your parents, your cousins, aunts and uncles, your spouse. *Ask your children.* Ask them all this question: "Were you ever molested?" Ask yourself.

The high instance of child sexual abuse in Utah, in active Mormon households by "priesthood" holders, crimes against children who grew up in the church then left the church, creates an ever-growing cast-away population. The Mormon church must claim it, or perish by societal fractures of its own making.

A note on the priesthood: All male Mormons 12 years or older, deemed worthy by church officials, can be "ordained" into the priesthood. Mormon women do not hold the priesthood. Priesthood holders – bishops, elders, high priests, priests and deacons – manage the church's business, worship activities and finances through an unpaid lay ministry set up by priesthood officials who call members to positions of authority after praying for guidance to make assignments.

Everybody Knows

Is there something in the water, the food or is everyone just desensitized and medicated? Everybody knows about the child molestation, the rapes, and the alarming numbers of each in Utah. People talk about it. *It's a matter of common knowledge.* Yet no one has sounded the alarm.

Most societies, religions and community groups protect and nurture their children. Not here. Some 96% of a random 500 persons I've talked with in four years knew about or have heard about the excessive number of child sexual assaults in this state. Just last week, I ran into a man who had been in Utah for a few months from his native Seattle. I asked him: "Have you heard about what they do to their children here?"

He didn't hesitate in his answer, "Yeah, they molest them." Two other people nearby, Utah natives, chimed in with details.

Let me point out, I have no secret anti-Mormon agenda. In fact, I've never been interested in Mormonism or Utah, in particular. I didn't set out to write this book. However, I am interested in people. And the epidemic of child sexual abuse in this area became quickly apparent – an honest observation that came to me after talking with people.

If the more than 70% of Utahns who claim Mormon standing actually adhered to the LDS principle of "family first," the state *should* have one of the lowest child sexual assault rates in the nation. This is not the case.

Utah ranks 8th highest in child sexual abuse incidents out of the 40 states reporting to the Child Welfare League of America, according to most recent statistics reported in 1998. Statistics show 2.6 children of every 1,000 in Utah were sexually molested or raped that year. A majority of state's reported *fewer than half that many* children per 1,000 being sexually abused. That means 1,823 of Utah's 701,300 children under 17 years old reported being sexually assaulted in 1998. The national average was 1.6 per 1,000 children.

The number of unreported instances is far greater, because victims are afraid to tell anyone what has happened, and the legal procedure for validating an incident is painstaking and seriously flawed. Health professionals estimate 1-in-4 girls and 1-in-6 boys will be sexually assaulted before the age of 18. These figures more accurately reflect the crisis in Utah. Many may think the numbers exaggerated. Sadly, from my research and interviews with Utahns molested as children, these statistics ring true. Still no one acknowledges the epidemic, let alone attempts to contain it. The church and state appear ill equipped to do so. It doesn't seem to be a priority at all.

Case in point: In July 2001, an elder of the Mormon church digitally (finger) raped a 4-year-old girl in a small, dark supply closet at the church while her mother met for about an hour with three priesthood leaders at a disciplinary council in the bishop's office. The "bishop's court" took place up the stairs only a few feet from the basketball gym where Elder Johnson had volunteered to watch the child. Lisa and her mother, Becky, will unfortunately never forget that day.

A few weeks later, a Salt Lake City child abuse detective interviewed Lisa alone in an enclosed room to record her disclosure on videotape. The detective looked so much like the perpetrator that they could pass for brothers. Lisa would not talk. When Becky mentioned this to the detective he said he saw no reason why his similar look and the fact he was a male stranger alone with Lisa in a small, unfamiliar room would make any difference in the outcome of the interview. This is the department's top child sexual abuse investigator? It's hard to believe but true.

No criminal charges were filed against Elder Johnson despite detailed testimony from Lisa and from at least six witnesses to whom she voluntarily disclosed this man's actions. (*Penetration with a finger of a child under 14 years of age is considered aggravated sexual abuse of a child, a first-degree felony punishable by five years to life in prison.*)

"Now my daughter has this memory, this life event, like some sick tattoo that cannot be erased," Becky says. "At least her protest of NO! against her abuser and her courage in telling will bring about a change. *Because I am shouting out the secret!* If there are predators in your midst lock them up, get them help and limit their access to your congregation, family and friends."

Abuse Is *Not* Simply "Touching"

In Utah, there exists this bizarre, pervasive, ingrained attitude that child sexual abuse "isn't that bad": *What is everybody getting so upset about? We know it's against the law but maybe it really shouldn't be. You know, it's just touching. Everyone has a rough childhood. It happens to all of us, doesn't it?*

This attitude has been expressed to me often by adults molested as children who simply want to "get on with" their lives. Molestation, rape and incest are minimized across the board. The mind-set is widely held by the victims' mothers and fathers, other family members and siblings, and by Mormon clergy and church members. I've heard horrendous cases of child sexual battery described as "touching," as if the experience is some kind of expected and accepted rite of passage. Even inappropriate "touching" is not acceptable in healthy societies.

Sexual abuse is molestation and rape, from inappropriate caressing and fondling to digital, object and penal penetration. Fondling sounds tame. Don't be deceived.

What these abusers do is rip into the victim's body and mind. Fondling becomes forced finger or object rape of the vagina and anus, invasive and often violent oral copulation, anal rape with the penis (sodomy), and painful, physically and psychologically destructive forced intercourse that may include beatings. Sexual abuse is so often, in reality, the bloody mutilation of a child.

Some predators, of course, will prime their child victims, not employing overt violence, and mold them into "lovers." This is an insidious and vicious form of rape. The victim associates abuse with love and pleasurable sexual feelings. These children not only lose their parent figure but the child/parent relationship becomes something else, something depraved, immoral and caustic. The victim is not a child and not an equal, but a slave to the pedophile's demented and selfish needs and desires. When the molester is a trusted friend, victims lose their ability to trust themselves and others.

This is often the harder cycle to break because it carries no apparent physical injury and is wrapped tightly in the seemingly soft blanket of "love" all the while lined with razors that trap the child victim, and in time the adult, in emotional and psychological paralysis. Don't move or you'll be cut to shreds.

Don't let anyone fool you. Child sexual abuse and incest is *always* a violent assault of its victims no matter whether the hand that hurts them employs a slap or a caress.

Oppression Fuels Abuse

I have comforted, cried with and counseled hundreds of children, women and men, as well as seniors in my professional and personal interactions. I know the pain of abuse is real. The long-term emotional and psychological damage of child sexual molestation, rape and incest is devastating.

As they mature, victims experience depression, anxiety, panic attacks, self-hate, fatigue, excessive sleep, drug addiction, sexual dysfunction, extreme rage, and eating disorders from self-starvation to chronic overeating that leads to severe obesity. Destructive behaviors arising from this history usually are passed on to the next generation if the victim does not undergo adequate individual or group therapy.

People ask, "How can you do that kind of work? Doesn't it get to you?" My job is working with people, it comes naturally to me. I am blessed with the insight, empathy and compassion that allow me to do what I do, and I love what I do. Where I'm from, there is ZERO tolerance for anyone who molests or rapes a child. I don't have a cloud of religious indoctrination hanging over me. So, I can see clearly: *From Utah to Zanzibar, it is socially suicidal and humanly immoral to molest and rape your own or anybody else's offspring.* I'm not intimidated nor impressed by child molesters. Their behavior should be punished and eradicated.

Why would a church that claims Christ-like values tolerate rampant abuse? My answer is this – *oppression fuels abuse.* The LDS church has deep racist, sexist and elitist roots, attitudes that still exist today. Here I want to give some information on the doctrinal discrimination and prejudice that treats people of color, women and children as second-class citizens in Mormon society.

Mormonism teaches that the black race is "inferior" and "cursed" by God. For the first 150 years the church existed, black men could not be initiated into the Mormon priesthood, although their money in tithing was welcomed.

Also for the first 60 years, the church said male members needed to marry multiple wives in order to enter into God's highest kingdom. Polygamy is nothing short of domestic slavery. The church only abandoned the practice after the United States government started throwing polygamists in jail. Mormon leaders who taught these things are revered by church members as "prophets, seers and revelators."

In June 1978, Mormon officials proclaimed that "worthy" black males could "hold the priesthood." This turnabout came as church leaders planned to initiate their final drive to send their "missionaries" into the remaining lands of the world where Mormonism had been most resisted – particularly Africa. Despite the change, the teaching that a race of people are "cursed with a black skin" for sins committed by them before they were born remains. No "revelation" has ever removed that long-held belief.

"Had I anything to do with the Negro, I would confine them by strict law to their own species and put them on a national equalization," said Joseph Smith, founder of the Mormon church. (*History of the Church,* Volume 5, pages 218-219.)

9

Second Mormon president Brigham Young said: "You see some classes of the human family that are *black, uncouth, uncomely, disagreeable, sad, low in their habits, wild, and seemingly without the blessings of the intelligence that is generally bestowed upon mankind.* The first man that committed the crime of killing one of his brethren will be cursed the longest. Cain slew his brother. This was not to be and the Lord put a mark on him, *which is the flat nose and black skin.*" (*Journal of Discourses*, Volume 7, pages 290-291)

Young also said death would be the penalty for interracial marriage and bearing biracial children: "Shall I tell you the law of God in regard to the African race? If the white man who belongs to the chosen seed mixes his blood with the seed of Cain, the penalty, under the law of God, is death on the spot. *This will always be so.*" (*Journal of Discourses,* Volume 10, page 110.)

Modern-day member of the LDS Quorum of Twelve Apostles, the late Bruce R. McConkie, said: "*The Negroes are not equal with other races when the receipt of spiritual blessings are concerned,* particularly the priesthood and the temple blessings. This inequality is not of man's origin. It is the Lord's doing, based on His eternal laws of justice, and *grows out of the lack of spiritual valiance of those concerned.*" (*Mormon Doctrine*, 10th printing, pages 527-528.) McConkie back-peddled after the 1978 decision: "Forget everything that I have said, or what Brigham Young or whosoever has said in days past that is contrary to the present revelation. We spoke with a limited understanding and without the light and knowledge that now has come into the world."

After then-LDS president Spencer W. Kimball announced the revelation, apostle LeGrand Richards attempted to explain the church's dramatic new position: "Down in Brazil, there is so much Negro blood in the population there that it's hard to get leaders that don't have Negro blood in them. We just built a temple down there. It's going to be dedicated in October. All those people with Negro blood in them have been raising the money to build that temple. If we don't change, then they can't even use it."

It seems the Mormon God comes through by changing his mind just about the same time financial gain or modern-day politics demand the church get with the program.

10

Almost An About Face

Quite recently, in 1998, the *Los Angeles Times,* quoting Mormon priesthood leaders, reported that the LDS church was considering disavowing past doctrine concerning the African race and that such an announcement would come soon.

Church officials later vehemently denied the report.

The *Times* article read in part: "Twenty years after the Mormon church dropped its ban against blacks in the priesthood, key leaders are debating a proposal to repudiate historic church doctrines that were used to bolster claims of black inferiority.

"The proposal to disavow the teachings, which purport to link African skin color to curses from God in Hebrew and Mormon scriptures, is under review by the LDS Committee on Public Affairs, made up of members of the church's general authorities.

"Although church leaders now proclaim racial equality as a *fundamental teaching*, repudiating old doctrine remains difficult. Those involved say leaders want to retract earlier statements without undermining the faith of believers. *They feel like a lot of people may not believe the church is true because a lot of these things were said by previous prophets, and a true prophet of God shouldn't make mistakes,* said David Jackson, an African American Mormon.

"Mormons, as well as other churches, have taught that Africans descended from the biblical personages Cain and Ham, who displeased God and were cursed. Over time, the curses came to be associated with black skin and used to justify slavery and, in the case of the Mormon church, for denying its priesthood to blacks. Mormon theology added another explanation: Blacks on Earth were among spirit children who failed to fight valiantly for God during a heavenly war with the devil. Nonetheless, they were permitted to take human form in black bodies. For that reason, the 1978 revelation shocked the Mormon world, and was widely celebrated as a new dispensation."

An African Origin

Unbelievable to me are the many Utahns who don't know of long-standing scientific research, backed by DNA evidence, that shows the human species originated in Africa. "Fossil evidence supports that modern humans appeared earliest in Africa," says anthropologist Chris Stringer, a scientist at the British Museum of Natural History in London.

"We can all trace our ancestry from Africa. We are all very closely related, American Indians, Australian Aborigines, Eskimos and Europeans. Under the skin, we are all Africans," he says.

Genetic research also traces human origins to Africa. Becky Cann, a geneticist at the University of Hawaii, has gathered evidence of one part of the DNA molecule that only females can pass on. She compared modern DNA samples with evidence from anthropological excavations in Africa. "All humans alive today can trace their ancestry in genes dating back to a single female who we think lived in Africa 200,000 years ago," Cann says.

Another fact rarely considered by white people in Utah is that the black race is the only race able to reproduce every color of person that exists on Earth, including white or albino. This indicates that all races originated from the African race. The African continent is the Mother Land – the first homeland from which human kind evolved. This information should bind us because we are all human beings arising from the same seed. We are human brothers and sisters, all equal under God. Mormons show scientific and spiritual ignorance when they claim God cursed the very people from whom they originated.

Even though the LDS church accepted the black man into its priesthood some 25 years ago, it seems the daily activities of the church, at least in Salt Lake City, still cannot accommodate people of color in a mainstream way. Can the Mormon of color walk into any one of the 16,000 LDS churches worldwide and feel at home? Apparently not. Little known to white Mormons in Utah, the church has set aside a congregation known as "Genesis" made up of mostly blacks, and interracial couples and families. They meet each Sunday in a small chapel in South Salt Lake.

Could this be the result of prejudice and bigotry that began when Brigham Young told his flock they would be struck down dead if they mixed with the African race?

Polygamy's Sick Legacy

From my research, I believe the LDS practice of polygamy has evolved into generations of sexually abused children who suffer in silence, shackled to a society that refuses to protect them. For more than six decades, the church preached and practiced polygamy as a spiritual law and prerequisite to reach the highest kingdom in Mormon heaven.

12

Mormon founder Joseph Smith had an estimated 30 wives, the youngest one being 14 years old when he had sex with her after a secret religious marriage ceremony. Smith was in his 30s. Historians report that Smith was also "sealed" to a 15-year-old girl and two 16-year-old girls. These marriages occurred when Smith was 37 and 38 years old, an adult victimizing children.

Smith and his followers were continually persecuted for their religious practices, especially that of having sexual relations with child brides. Outraged citizens drove Mormons from New York State to Ohio, then to Missouri and Illinois, and finally across the plains to Utah. Chiefly because of polygamist activity, Smith was killed in 1844 when a mob attacked him in the Carthage jail where he was being held on charges of treason after the governor of Illinois ordered firearms of the Mormon militia be turned over. Just before his arrest, Smith led the destruction of a Nauvoo, Illinois, newspaper that had printed information on his "secret sexual liaisons" and multiple wives.

After Smith's death, Brigham Young became the second president of the LDS church and led some 30,000 Mormons out of Nauvoo in February 1846. Pioneers arrived in what would become the Salt Lake Valley on July 24, 1847. Historical accounts report that when Young saw the land, he said: "This is the right place."

Young had 55 wives, 16 of whom bore him 57 children.

From its inception until today, the Mormon church has had a deceptive partnership with polygamy. At first, in 1835, the church denied practicing polygamy, then publicly embraced it in 1843 and finally, by law, officially abolished the practice in 1890 after an ultimatum from the United States government.

In the first edition of the Mormon book of scripture known as the *Doctrine & Covenants* printed in 1835, the church denounced polygamy: *"Inasmuch as this church of Christ has been reproached with the crime of fornication, and polygamy: we declare that we believe, that one man should have one wife; and one woman, but one husband, except in the case of death, when either is at liberty to marry again."* (*Doctrine and Covenants*, Section 101, verse 4)

This denial was printed in the *Doctrine & Covenants* until the year 1876. At that time, the Mormon leaders inserted Section 132, which permits and even encourages plural marriage. To have one section condemn polygamy and another approve it would be contradictory, so the original was removed from scripture.

Section 132 reads in part: "For behold, I reveal unto you a new and an everlasting covenant; and if ye abide not that covenant, then are ye damned; for no one can reject this covenant and be permitted to enter into my glory." Several versus explain that Mormons must marry in the temple "for time and all eternity" in order for the union to continue after death. Then the writings detail the "law" of plural marriage.

"Abraham received promises concerning his seed . . . and as touching Abraham and his seed, out of the world they should continue as innumerable as the stars . . . This promise is yours also. Go ye, therefore and do the works of Abraham, enter into my law and ye shall be saved. God commanded Abraham, and Sarah gave Hagar to Abraham to wife. Because this was the law; and from Hagar sprang many people . . . And again, as pertaining to the law of the priesthood – *if any man espouse a virgin, and the first give her consent, and if he espouse the second, then is he justified; he cannot commit adultery for they are given him; for he cannot commit adultery with that that belongeth unto him and to no one else. And if he have ten virgins given unto him by this law, he cannot commit adultery, for they belong to him; therefore is he justified."*

It seems the Lord also had a message for Smith's wife: "And I command mine handmaid, Emma Smith, to abide and cleave unto my servant, Joseph, and to none else. But if she will not abide this commandment she shall be destroyed saith the Lord; for I am the Lord thy God, and will destroy her if she abide not in my law."

Section 132 arose from a revelation God supposedly gave to Joseph Smith on July 12, 1843. *That same year, Smith told the press that Mormons did not practice polygamy.* By that time, Smith himself had married 12 women, taking a 17-year-old orphan as his second wife in 1835.

Young said that in order for a man to be exalted in the afterlife, he must be a polygamist: "The only men who become gods, even the Sons of God, are those who enter into polygamy." (*Journal of Discourses*, Vol. 11, page 269)

Heber C. Kimball, second counselor to Brigham Young, said monogamy would prematurely age a man: "I have noticed that a man who has but one wife soon begins to wither and dry up, while a man who goes into plurality looks fresh, young and sprightly. Why is this? Because God loves that man and he honors his word. *For a man of god to be confined to one woman is a small business. I do not know what we should do if we had only one wife apiece."* (*Deseret News*, April 1857.)

14

Though polygamy is no longer practiced in mainstream Mormonism, many fundamentalist Mormons, who broke away from the church, do still take more than one wife. Reports estimate from as few as 30,000 to as many as 100,000 polygamists living within the state of Utah.

Even today's mainstream Mormonism does not completely distance itself from polygamy. Smith's revelation calling for polygamy still is published as scripture. Active LDS members believe that polygamy will be practiced in the afterlife by men who themselves plan to be gods and fathers of eternal families. The LDS church teaches that worthy men, after they die, will be exalted to the "celestial kingdom" on a planet called "Kolob" (no kidding, they really teach this) where God the Father resides and will tutor polygamist priesthood holders to be gods themselves. These men will need a multitude of wives to procreate spirit children who will in turn be given bodies and live their mortal lives on other Earth-like planets.

As part of the marriage ceremony in LDS temples, the man is allowed to know his wife's temple or secret name. He will call this name to bring his eternal mate(s) into their celestial destination. Interestingly enough, the woman is not allowed to know her husband's temple name. Mormon men can marry or be "sealed" to more than one woman during a lifetime (for example, if his first wife dies and he marries a subsequent wife in the temple.) Women cannot be sealed to more than one husband.

As an example of national concerns about how Utah handles polygamy, consider this *City Weekly* article written by associate editor Ben Fulton and published Jan. 31, 2002: "The National Organization for Women compares Utah's fundamentalist Mormon polygamists to Afghanistan's Taliban: *The Taliban and the polygamist commit domestic violence in innumerable ways using rape, bondage, servitude, incest, trafficking in girls, forced marriages and subservience to men as a way of life.* Charles R. Castle, executive vice president with a NOW political action committee in California, said: 'NOW was formed to eliminate slave and master laws. You have polygamists showing up at Utah State Capitol meetings. In any other state, these people would be arrested. We find the selective enforcement of the law an outrage.'

"In 1998, a 16-year-old girl phoned 911 after a belt-whipping from her polygamist father because she refused to be the 15th wife to her uncle. The incident exposed Salt Lake's Kingston polygamy clan.

"In June 1999, David Ortell Kingston was convicted of having sexual relations with his teenage niece. Just last August, polygamist Tom Green, who married two of his wives when they were 14, was sentenced to five years in prison on felony bigamy and criminal non-support. Green still faces a felony charge for rape of a child," after fathering the son of his 13-year-old stepdaughter in 1986.

"In 2000, the Utah House voted down a bill targeting the crimes of incest, sexual abuse and tax fraud among polygamists because some lawmakers said it smacked of hate-crime discrimination."

Harboring Sexual Predators

Utah laws and church policies do not protect children. The Mormon church claims child sexual abuse is no more prevalent in the church than in the general public, and that the church is working to help victims. Facts of recent cases and official comments from church leaders show just the opposite is true.

On March 9, 2001, the Utah Supreme Court banned lawsuits seeking compensation over LDS clergy malpractice. The landmark ruling grants broad protections to church leaders when they hear of sexual abuse allegations against members. The high court unanimously upheld a trial judge's decision to dismiss a child rape victim's lawsuit against the church. The reason for the decision cited First Amendment safeguards against government intrusion into religious practices. The lawsuit filed by Lynette Franco claimed her bishop and stake president were negligent by ignoring her pleas for help after she told them, when she was 7 years old, she had been sexually abused by a teenage church member.

Justice Leonard Russon said the court did not define a standard of practice for LDS clergy because "that would embroil the courts in establishing the training, skill and standards applicable for members of the clergy in this state in a diversity of religions professing widely varying beliefs." All five justices of Utah's Supreme Court are Mormon.

LDS church spokesman, Dale Bills, in a press release said: *"The decision preserves religious liberty and freedom for all and confirms that lawsuits like these have no merit. We regret that Lynette Earl Franco and her family are unhappy with the church and hope that they can find peace."*

This is patronizing, condescending, hypocritical and immoral. Clergy should serve and protect their members. The men who heard the victim's plea must accept responsibility for their failure to help this child. They may have been the only ones to know she was being victimized and their inaction guaranteed this little girl would continue to be molested by a member of the church. Religious freedom, even under Utah's Constitution, but especially under the Constitution of the United States, does *not* include the freedom to harbor pedophiles. LDS church officials better hope that *they* can find peace through God's grace. How can anyone on Earth forgive this travesty?

Franco's attorney Ed Montgomery, as quoted in the *Salt Lake Tribune*, said: "This ruling means the LDS church is completely immune from anything they do behind closed doors. It's chilling, is what it is. The most powerful organization in this state is doing what it will, without any government regulation, and without any redress available." Montgomery said his clients are considering an appeal to the United States Supreme Court.

Linda Walker, director of *Child Protection Project* in Oakland, California, wrote to the *Tribune* editor: "Every Mormon beware of the nice man from church assigned as your home teacher, primary teacher, or Scout leader. He just got his *get-out-of-jail-free* card from the all-Mormon Supreme Court. The pedophile underground already cites Utah as a very safe haven for them, with lax child protection laws and enforcement. I'm certain many pedophiles have already hopped a bus to Temple Square. LDS spokesman Dale Bills can baptize them. As for me, I'm throwing up."

Maybe church authorities will start to take charges of sexual abuse seriously when their inaction cuts into their pocketbook as it did recently in Oregon. The church settled for $3 million after a family sued saying Mormon authorities knew of a pedophile's history and did not tell them before they let him into their home.

On Sept. 5, 2001, *The Oregonian* reported: "The Mormon church announced a $3 million settlement of a sex-abuse case brought by a Portland man abused as a boy by a high priest. Alleging negligence, Jeremiah Scott's lawsuit accused the church of knowingly allowing a child molester access to children. In his 1998 lawsuit, Scott said the church hid the fact that Franklin Richard Curtis, one of its high priests, was a pedophile.

"Curtis had been excommunicated in 1983 in Pennsylvania but was re-baptized in 1984 in Michigan. In 1988, he joined the Brentwood Ward in Portland. Curtis lived with the Scott family twice, in 1990 and 1991, at Scott's parents' invitation. He repeatedly abused Scott on the second stay. At the time, Curtis was 87 and Scott was 11. Curtis was later convicted of sex abuse.

"Scott's mother, Sandra Scott, had consulted her bishop, Gregory Lee Foster, about taking Curtis in. Foster advised her that she shouldn't because of his advanced age but said nothing about pedophilia, although he knew of complaints about Curtis. Foster testified that he didn't remember the complaints against Curtis at the time of his conversation with Sandra Scott. The bishop later admitted that he knew Curtis' past but didn't tell Scott because Curtis had repented of his crimes."

World Beware!

Little boys as young as 3 in the Mormon church know the song by heart: *"I hope they call me on a mission when I have grown a foot or two. I hope to be a missionary to work and teach and preach like missionaries do."* This is one reason the rest of the world might want to know Utah's dirty "little" secret.

It is a fact most people who perpetuate sex crimes were once victims themselves. This decadent cycle of behaviors has a seriously profound effect on a large number of people around the world because – while the LDS church turns a deaf ear to the multitudes of victims of sex crimes, it continues to churn out thousands of missionaries every year. In 2000, the church sent out 61,000 full-time missionaries around the world and baptized a reported 274,000 converts. These teenage missionaries leave their homes with tons of emotional baggage to be unleashed on unsuspecting families searching for religious identity.

Mormons believe that every male at age 19 should volunteer to serve an unpaid two-year mission to preach LDS doctrine. Missionaries work together in twos as roommates, study partners and teaching companions who preach church lessons throughout neighborhoods. These young men, who usually travel by foot or bicycle, are commonly seen to be fresh faced, neatly dressed in dark suits with crisp white shirts and dark ties. They adhere to highly disciplined schedules and teaching goals. They cannot go to movies, listen to music or watch television.

The missionaries may themselves be too new in their religious development to know what they believe or to have a fixed independent belief, yet they have been taught and they teach that the Mormon church is the "only true church." These young men are pushed together in close quarters at a sensitive time in their lives, emotionally, religiously and sexually. LDS church doctrine forbids homosexual behavior and masturbation, but the nature of the situation places these youths at risk for being victims and/or perpetrators of sexual abuse.

The social pressure to serve a Mormon mission is intense. Young women in search of a husband to marry in the temple usually date *only* returned missionaries. Non-missionaries are not popular choices in the social circles of Mormon young adults.

Mormons do allow women to serve missions at age 21 if they are not yet married. Marriage is encouraged in young adulthood even before either gender finishes post high school job training or college. Birth control in marriage is discouraged. Mormon couples are encouraged to have as many children as they can afford as soon and as often as possible.

Mormons who voluntarily have sex before marriage are socially branded. They must go through a process of repentance and discipline which may include disfellowship (by which they can attend church and pay tithing but not take part in religious rituals.) Sometimes the person will be excommunicated before he or she can be re-baptized and marry in the temple.

Virginity for marriageable Mormons is such a must that during early sexual experimentation and especially for victims of childhood abuse, oral sex is not considered "real" sex by a great number of young church members. Thus, many of the safety measures – such as abstaining from oral sex – that protect youngsters from being molested by adolescents and adults are compromised at an early age. Victims reported to me that they were forced to perform oral sex on adult parental figures or older siblings for much of their young lives thus conditioning them for further dysfunctional sexual development into adulthood.

Inadequate sex education also negatively impacts a Mormon's sexual development. LDS parents have consistently lobbied against sex education in schools. The education in homes is sorely lacking, most of the time stressing abstinence only and prohibiting masturbation.

19

When pre-adolescents and adolescents are told they cannot masturbate, how do they handle natural physiological needs and desires? If they masturbate and are made to feel deeply guilty about the activity, then they have no healthy release. What happens? Their sexual activities are pushed underground, into secret liaisons and aberrant behavior, sometimes as victims of demented adults or as abusers of children who do not tell.

When boys and girls grow up like this, what is to become of their adult sexual relationships within marriage? They take no education and no experience into the bedroom. No wonder so many LDS couples complain of unsatisfactory sex. They know little about their partner's sexuality or even the workings of their own bodies. Women often don't know how to come to orgasm because they had to keep their hands off themselves. Many Mormon men don't know how to bring a woman to orgasm.

The church discourages married couples from engaging in oral sex with each other. If this is a strong desire of one partner or another, where does he or she go to meet that need? Again, they cannot masturbate. If a person does not have the spiritual and physical freedom to express healthy, normal sexual desires within an adult relationship – then children will suffer when these adults turn to trusting, quiet victims for satisfaction.

The Mormon Olympics

The biggest Mormon missionary effort took place in Salt Lake City during the 2002 Winter Olympic Games. The city had an estimated 700,000 or more visitors, about 9,000 journalists and worldwide television coverage.

On Jan. 28, 2002, *The Washington Post* reported how pervasive the LDS church was in the games: "To counter the *Mormon Olympics* image, Gordon B. Hinckley, the church's 91-year-old president, has declared that missionaries will not buttonhole potential converts during the Games here next month. The word from on high is: Keep a low, polite, neighborly profile. Show the world that the Latter-day Saints are a wholesome, vibrant, conservative but mainstream Christian religion and not some weird cult of polygamists.

"There is really no other place in America where one religion so dominates daily life. The role of the Mormon faith in Utah is often compared, favorably, to Catholicism in Rome and Judaism in Israel, or unfavorably by its critics, to Islamic theocracies in the Middle East.

20

"The head of the Salt Lake Organizing Committee, Mitt Romney, is a Mormon bishop. The two leaders of the bidding team who brought the Games to the city – and scandal, too, because of their enticements to the International Olympic Committee – are also Mormons. Ditto the governor, the entire congressional delegation and the overwhelming majority of Utah's judges, mayors, city councils, school boards and state legislators. All downtown addresses are numbered by their distance from the temple. Mormons own one of the city's two daily newspapers as well as the local NBC television affiliate and radio stations."

Maybe president Hinckley's mandate for missionaries to keep a low profile had nothing to do with trying to accommodate visitors and not bother them. Mormon leaders know that the international media is in town, and journalists tend to ask detailed, rigorous and often uncomfortable questions.

A few things Mormons may not want the world to know:

Religious rituals take place in 124 expensive, elaborately ornate LDS temples throughout the world. The secret activities meant only for worthy, active members include:
- baptisms for the dead
- washings and anointings
- hand signals that depict how a member will have the "throat cut, breast cut open, and bowels torn out" if he or she reveals temple secrets
- secret tokens, signals, symbols and words or chants that priesthood members must know to enter God's kingdom

Priesthood members use secret handshakes. They employ certain knuckle and finger positions during a handshake, even outside the church and the temple, so they can tell who is a "friend or foe" of the Mormon church.

Temple-worthy individuals wear special underwear, called garments. Mormons claim the garments protect them from physical harm. Garments for both men and women extend over the shoulders and just below the knee. The garments open at the crotch. Small symbols mark the nipples, navel and right knee. The church encourages husband and wife to wear the garments during sexual intercourse.

21

God resides on planet Kolob. When worthy Mormons die they will join God on this planet, located in the Cancerian constellation, where they will learn how to become gods.

God the Father was once a man. He progressed in learning and experience to become a God. God also has a perfect, tangible body of flesh and bone. Jesus has the same.

God had sex with Mary. Jesus Christ was not born of a virgin. According to LDS teachings, the savior of humankind was "begotten by an Immortal Father in the same way that mortal men are begotten by mortal fathers." (*Mormon Doctrine*, p.547)

You must be Mormon to be saved. "If it had not been for Joseph Smith and the restoration, there would be no salvation. There is no salvation outside the Church of Jesus Christ of Latter-day Saints." (*Mormon Doctrine*, p. 670)

The Garden of Eden was in Missouri. "The early brethren of this dispensation taught that the Garden of Eden was located in the land of Zion, an area for which Jackson County, Missouri, is the center place." (*Mormon Doctrine*, p. 20)

I will explore Mormon beliefs and doctrine in more detail in *Chapter 4: LDS Sacred Or Sordid Secrets?* Now, let me share with you the heart-breaking story of a 4-year-old molested just months ago by a Mormon priesthood holder. This case is all too typical and happens daily in LDS churches and homes.

Chapter 2

This Is What They Do Here

Her mother calls her Lisa Lightenin' Bug because this child glows. Her energy is contagious and she, like most toddlers, has a unique perspective on the world.

One day Lisa was climbing her way up her mother's back as Mom sat exhausted against the couch. Exasperated, Becky huffed at her daughter: "Lisa, what are you doing?"

"I'm climbing to the sky, Mama!"

In July 2001, Lisa's light dimmed. The little girl took on a disturbing shadow. She lashed out in uncontrollable tantrums, she clung on her mother and whined. Potty trained for a year, she began to wet herself. Then, Lisa told her mother that her "privates" hurt. She would cry in pain when she urinated. She would try to avoid going to the bathroom as long as possible. Her vaginal area was red, tender and irritated. Becky suspected that something terrible had happened to her child when she was not around to protect her.

"I asked Lisa right away, if anyone touched her private area. She seemed upset and just kept saying, *No, no, no,*" Becky says. "I tried to check out every possible reason for her physical discomfort and troubled behavior."

Lisa was proud of being tough like a *Power Puff* girl before then. "Suddenly, she was having nightmares and didn't want me to turn off the lights or shut the door to her bedroom," her mom says. "She started saying, *Mama, don't leave me!*"

Becky took Lisa to the doctor who also questioned the little girl about possible molestation, asking if specific adult males in her circle or anyone at daycare had touched her. Lisa said "no" to each inquiry. The checkup showed irritation but no noticeable trauma to the vagina. For about four more weeks, Lisa's behavior and physical complaints continued to be a mystery.

One Sunday night in late July, Becky became frightened and alarmed. This time Lisa didn't whine about her privates hurting, she shouted out in pain! Becky checked her daughter's private area and discovered the tissue from *the inside of Lisa's vagina was red and swollen, protruding about a fourth of an inch to the outside of the very small vaginal opening.* This was not a common irritation or usual injury to a toddler's privates, Becky knew this. But she didn't know what to do. In hindsight, she realized she should have taken Lisa directly to the emergency room. Instead, she wrapped ice in a washcloth and applied it to the area to bring the swelling down and numb her daughter's pain. The next day, Becky scheduled another appointment with Lisa's doctor.

A Trusted Friend?

Elder Johnson takes care of the church building, opens and locks the doors when there are functions going on. He is the self-designated daycare person, taking care of the members' children when they might act up during meetings. He's well known especially to single mothers looking for some peace so they can attend Sunday classes. This church has a higher number of single moms because it falls within the boundaries of a domestic violence safe house and a state-funded transitional housing complex for single parents.

Becky and Lisa moved into the housing complex and began attending the nearby Mormon church in April 2000.

Elder Johnson came with the missionaries to visit Becky and her daughter. He sat out on the porch with Lisa as her mother waved at them through the large living room window while she talked with the missionaries. At church, Elder Johnson would take the active and talkative Lisa into the hall or foyer during Sunday worship service (called "sacrament" meeting) so her mother could pay attention to the speakers. At times, he also took Lisa to the nursery or children's "primary" class while her mother attended Sunday school and an hour-long meeting for Relief Society, the women's auxiliary of the Mormon church.

After a few months when the six missionary lessons or "discussions" ended, Elder Johnson continued to visit Becky and Lisa each week bringing by used toys or extra bread he'd gotten from the church. Only having her stay-at-home mom for a playmate, Lisa enjoyed Elder Johnson's attention. Due to health problems, Becky would sometimes lie down in the next room to rest while Elder Johnson watched videos with Lisa.

Spotting The Predator

I was present at the park in July when Lisa had one of her tantrums. She was wild-eyed, lost in rage she could not control, lashing out, arms and legs flailing, as her mother held her and tried to calm her. Lisa was verbally repetitious as she fixated (two-word) sentences and did not respond to verbal redirection. From my experience, her behavior reminded me of a child acting out after being traumatized.

Sometime in August, completely by coincidence, I met Elder Johnson and observed his interaction with Lisa. Pretending to be reading, I peeked under the bill of my ball cap and watched as he played with her. He seemed territorial and too intimate. His touches were more like caresses than tickles. Something wasn't right. I knew he wasn't right.

I asked Becky about Elder Johnson and she seemed to trust him. However, there were obviously some institutional controls at work since she was raised in the church and was a victim of child sexual abuse herself. She had been conditioned and oriented to certain controls – social, religious and domestic. Since my radar went up, I decided to do some investigating on my own.

Becky's friend across the hall also knew Elder Johnson so I asked her about him. The Mormon neighbor said she was uncomfortable with how Elder Johnson acted around her own teenage son. "I have a real bad feeling about him!" she said. "He gives me the creeps!" We spoke a little longer about specific behaviors she had observed in Elder Johnson.

I talked with Lisa's mother again and shared my concerns.

The next day on their way to daycare, Becky asked Lisa about Elder Johnson. "Lisa was in her car seat in the back and I just looked at her casually through the rearview mirror when we stopped at a light," Becky says. "Lisa, has Elder Johnson ever touched you?" Lisa's face froze. Without hesitation she said, "Yes, mama, Elder Johnson put his finger in my privates and hurt me!" Then she began to sob.

"I really didn't expect that answer," Becky says. "My heart just dropped. I knew she was telling me what really happened. She wouldn't know that detail. She wouldn't know that it hurt unless he did this to her!" Becky went to Child Protective Services and reported him. A CPS worker interviewed Lisa and became convinced beyond a doubt that Elder Johnson molested this child. She encouraged Becky to take her complaint to police.

As more details came to light, investigators discovered that while Becky was in a disciplinary council or "court" with the bishop of her congregation and two other Mormon priesthood officials, Elder Johnson took her 4-year-old daughter to a supply closet and molested her. Then three weeks later, when Becky attended Sunday school class, Elder Johnson offered to take Lisa to the children's class. They never made it. Instead, once again, he took little Lisa to the supply closet and raped her with his finger: *"If you tell anyone, your mom will be mad at you! Do not tell your mom. She's mean. She will leave you!"*

When Elder Johnson hurt her, Lisa says, "I said, NO! really loud." Elder Johnson said, *"I love you."*

In his many years at the church, Elder Johnson must have had a field day. Babies by the dozen! As many as he wanted. Threatening to kill their moms if they told, scaring the hell out of these poor frightened children, many of whom are not old enough to speak and cannot even tell their story.

26

Child Protective Services held an administrative hearing in January to decide whether Elder Johnson can work with children in any state capacity. (No decision had been made at the time of publication of this book.) The outcome, however, won't restrict his access to children at church. After Becky took her complaint to her bishop, he "released" Elder Johnson from his "calling" as facilities manager which meant he lost the keys to the church and his open access to the building. However, church officials took no disciplinary action. Elder Johnson continues to hold the priesthood and can attend the temple as a "worthy" member.

The state refused to prosecute Elder Johnson who had other complaints against him prior to this one. As it looks, he has gotten away with rape. He's a felon on the streets.

"Some people I've talked to think this is not that serious," Becky says. "They think like, *oh, he touched her between the legs, big deal?* Come on! How does someone rape a 4-year-old? If he uses his penis, he'll kill her. So, he uses his finger. To a tiny girl, that's rape. This man raped my baby."

Lisa is undergoing therapeutic counseling and self-defense training. She is responding well considering. Five months after being raped by Elder Johnson, this brave child is again verbally pointing the finger at the pedophile. She mentioned him three times this month without prompting: "Elder Johnson hurt me!" She still goes through nights when she wakes up terrified, crying for her mother. She is still afraid at times to go into confined areas like the bathroom or near closets alone. But she is gaining power. Lisa says, "If Elder Johnson tries to hurt my privates again, I will stick him in the eye with my pencil!"

Note To The Honorable Elder Johnson: Are you reading this you pervert? We sent you a signed copy. This book is for Lisa Lightenin' Bug and all of Utah's children who have fallen prey to the likes of you.

God Is Not In It

Becky talked to me in detail about the social pressure to stay within the Mormon church even when it consistently abuses you. Like a battered spouse returning once again to an abusive partner, the victim feels compelled to give it one more try. Becky began re-investigating the church after she left her atheist husband in January 2000.

Becky thought if she started living the way she had been indoctrinated since she was a child, she would find peace and have a less chaotic life. Becky sought a cure to her troubles by revisiting exactly where the disease lived. Lying dormant for years, when she became active again in the church, the sickness awakened and infected her own daughter. She discovered that the solution she hoped for, Mormonism, was instead the problem.

She tells it best herself: "I grew up in the church. The pressure to conform is great. Most of my family members are Mormon and I care for them deeply. But the church is not for me. Even before Lisa was assaulted, I knew that. I just didn't want to accept that I didn't believe the Mormon religion.

"Through the years, I've learned that Mormons don't have a corner on the market of spirituality. You can be non-Mormon and have standards and values. Believe it or not, non-Mormons do have the power of prayer, of healing, of personal revelation and spiritual insight. When you've grown up in the church, and the church is all you know, it's difficult to understand that. I'm taking my name and Lisa's off the roles of the Church of Jesus Christ of Latter-day Saints. This, to many Mormons, means I have rejected my testimony and will perish in outer darkness or hell after my death. I know God doesn't work that way.

"Really, a church with this much power and money is suspect to me. Absolute power corrupts absolutely. When an establishment has a continuing problem with child sexual abuse and refuses to own up to and extinguish that epidemic, it has lost its connection with a Heavenly Father."

Becky continues: "I have to tell you it is a delight to discover the joyful noise – in song and testimony – others make when worshiping God. The Mormon church is stifling beyond belief. The meetings are dry and pedantic. Sacrament meeting is not so much about worshiping God and singing his praises, as it is about damaged people trying to find their way, or self-absorbed members trying to impress other members with their knowledge, wisdom and spiritual authority.

"Every Mormon woman knows the intense pressure to be perfect: To have a perfectly clean home, to raise perfectly mannered children, to have a perfectly attractive body, to have a perfectly successful husband.

28

"And if you are poor, you must *not* be living true principles of the gospel because God blesses the faithful with monetary success. Keeping up with the LDS culture is an enormous task. Women keep track of their family's religious accomplishments as if the record is a personal report card. To many Mormons, church activity is not seen as humble service, but as a status symbol – a never-ending cycle of religious elitism and climbing the social ladder to exaltation.

"I'm sure that many Mormons feel the church will help them avoid serious problems, keep trouble away and shelter them from disappointment. Maybe that is true for some people and Mormonism is a blessing to them. For me, the church has only caused more heartache in my life."

Believe The Children

This is what they do in Utah. They rape and molest little girls and boys. They ruin lives. They cause horrible nightmares and unimaginable pain to victims and families in extreme numbers. This is what they have done, this is what they're doing and what they will continue to do unless people who care about Utah's children come together to say, *"Oh, hell NO! No more!"*

Here are some myths about child sexual abuse that everyone should know and dispel:

MYTH: A child will make up stories of sexual abuse. Children rarely lie about being abused. These children are telling the truth. If anything, most children who are assaulted, don't tell at all.

MYTH: If the child doesn't report the abuse, run away or fight back, it can't be that bad. A child can love an abusive adult and crave his or her attention, even if it hurts. Children often think the abuse is "normal." They don't know anything else. Children know they can't survive on their own and don't want to jeopardize family support or friendships. Some think they won't be believed.

MYTH: Child sexual abuse only involves physical contact between the child and the abuser. Sexual abuse can include indecent exposure, crude talk about sex designed to shock the child or spark interest, indecent photographs of children, and forcing or allowing a child to watch sexual acts or materials.

MYTH: Children encourage abuse by acting seductive. No. Today's society encourages children to dress and act in a manner beyond their years. These children aren't looking for sex; they're just trying to fit in. *Any abuse is entirely the adult's responsibility.*

MYTH: Children are abused by strangers, like someone who stops to give them a ride to school. The majority of victims of child sexual assault are abused by parents, step-parents, siblings, other relatives or friends of the family. Stranger danger is real but children should be taught how to protect themselves from all dangerous people including friends and relatives.

MYTH: Children are resilient; they'll get over it. The effects of molestation, rape and incest on a child are serious and long lasting. They might include behavioral problems, depression, anxiety, eating disorders, confusion about sexual identity, nightmares and trouble sleeping. Some of these signs may not be obvious until the child becomes an adult.

Children who are abused also have trouble forming close relationships due to a loss of trust. The victim may need professional help to get over feelings of guilt and shame to realize that he or she is not to blame for the abuse. Victims of child sexual abuse may also have to deal with physical problems brought on by the assaults. They may have injuries of the genital area and reproductive system, painful urination or stomachaches, gastro-intestinal problems including diarrhea and constipation, and sexually transmitted diseases. Female victims who have reached puberty at the time of the abuse risk pregnancy.

Always victims must deal with emotional and psychological problems that share the stage with sexual abuse. Most employ self-destructive behaviors. Some may feel they should pay for their involvement in the abuse. They feel worthless and unlovable which can affect their schooling or work and disrupt relationships. Victims of child sexual abuse can develop dysfunctional attitudes toward sex, and it may be difficult for them to find satisfaction in a healthy sexual relationship later in life. They may turn to sexual acting out, prostitution or abuse of alcohol or other drugs. They may attempt or commit suicide.

30

Isn't It About Time?

Progressive and educated individuals of the white-male patriarchal power structure in the Church of Jesus Christ of Latter-day Saints need to speak out strongly and boldly. They must take swift action against child molesters to protect the innocence of Utah's children. The frightening part is these leaders already know of the epidemic, and have known for generations, of this evil cycle. Ignored, tolerated or dealt with incompetently, the disease has continued to grow in its scope and severity. To me, tolerance of evil is the same as giving permission, the same as encouraging this evil to continue – it becomes religiously sanctioned rape!

What can *you* do to prevent child sexual abuse?

As a parent:

- Know where your children are, who they are with and what they are doing.
- Ask your children what happens when they're alone with baby sitters, relatives and friends.
- Encourage your children to talk to you about *any* problems or questions they have.
- Talk with your children often every day about everyday things. Don't wait until there is a problem to talk.
- Teach your children to protect themselves and to set limits and boundaries concerning their personal space, who touches them and how.
- Teach them basic self-defense techniques.
- Teach them they can say "NO!" to anyone who does anything to them that makes them feel uncomfortable.
- If someone hurts them or attempts to molest them, tell your children to shout, scream, yell, kick, punch, and run away continuing to scream until they find help. They need to make a lot of noise and be heard.
- Tell them they do not have to please everyone they meet. Encourage them to develop an internal value system and openly share their own opinions and beliefs.
- Give them responsibilities that promote self-discipline, self-control and self-esteem. Do not be their servant. Let them learn to take care of and stand up for themselves.

As a member of your community:

- Report child abuse when you hear about it or suspect it. If you suspect abuse in Utah, call 1-800-678-9366.
- Pressure police to take more child sexual abuse reports to the District Attorney and make sure these perpetrators go to trial to answer charges against them.
- Lobby lawmakers to pass tougher laws demanding prison terms for child molesters and rapists.
- Encourage mandatory mental health treatment for accused and convicted child molesters.
- Demand the state prosecute incest just as it does "stranger" rape.
- Talk to your church leaders to make sure there is a plan in place that supports and protects victims of sexual abuse.
- Support children's rights to accurate information about sexual abuse and access to basic sex education.

What are parents and other adults to do when they are members of a church that allows child molesters and rapists to walk free and abuse children again and again? *Wake up!*

You don't have to keep following flawed attitudes and policies. Don't wait passively in line like a lamb to the slaughter. Get your children out of that line! You do have power. You can be instrumental in eradicating this immoral behavior. Each of you can make a difference. *Speak out and demand change.* Ignorance is not an excuse. Now, you know.

Chapter 3

Victims Tell The Secret:
Child Sexual Abuse Case Histories

What follows are true accountings of some of the hundreds of thousands of little girls, boys, adolescents, women and men who have been molested and raped in Utah. The stories are graphic, often described in vulgar language by the survivors. They are hard to read. I leave these accounts intact in order for the reader to fully realize the degenerate legacy that Male Mormon Molesters (3Ms) leave to their victims.

LDS children are indoctrinated from birth that masturbation and sexual intercourse before marriage are serious sins. Imagine the profound and lasting psychological injury that occurs when these children are molested and raped by the same Mormon "priesthood" holders who claim to be able to act with God's authority and power on Earth?

Victims of child sexual abuse in the Mormon church must battle deep-seated guilt and shame when they fail to protect their own chastity even when it is taken from them by force. Some victims believe death is a better alternative. In fact, the church has told them as much:

"There is no true Latter-day Saint who would not rather bury a son or a daughter than to have him or her lose his or her chastity – realizing that chastity is of more value than anything else in all the world," said the late LDS church president Heber J. Grant. (*The Miracle of Forgiveness*, by Spencer W. Kimball)

According to revered Mormon apostle Bruce R. McConkie: *"Loss of virtue is too great a price to pay even for preservation of one's life – better dead clean, than alive unclean."*

Suicides in Utah are more than *six times* the homicide rate. In 1999, 14.7 Utahns per 100,000 killed themselves, while only 2.4 per 100,000 people died by someone else's hand.

Utah ranks 9th highest among all 50 states in the number of suicides, according to National Vital Statistics Report for 1999. Why are Utahns killing themselves in such extreme numbers? The state's suicide rate is nearly 1.5 times the national rate of 10 per 100,000 people (30,575 suicides across the country.) Suicide is ranked as the 3rd highest killer among 15 to 24 year olds in the United States.

CAUTION: If you have the slight bit of concern that reading these accounts might trigger memories or difficult feelings concerning your own experience of child sexual abuse, please have the telephone number of a mental health crisis line on hand. Then follow up with an appointment with a counselor who works with adults molested as children.

3M = Male Mormon Molester

Janet, Case 01
Daddy's Girl: A 39-year-old white female, eldest and only girl of four children, who was 14 years old when she was first molested by her Mormon father, a respected Salt Lake City car dealer. Janet was 18 when this 3M fully raped her. The last sexual assault was a few months ago, Christmas 2001. Janet's mother has known all the while of her husband's crimes. In fact, the sickness goes so deep that Janet still associates with her parents as if nothing has happened. She grew up in West Jordan in the Salt Lake Valley.

Deon, Case 02
Perverted Parents: A 27-year-old white mother of two whose LDS parents have raped her all of her life. They also molested Deon's 4-year-old daughter who was finally rescued by her biological father. Deon now has a 3-month-old girl. Sadly, she and the baby live with her parents. She's from Salt Lake City.

Becky, Case 03
Step Monster: A 40-year-old white Mormon female molested from 6 to 17 years old by her stepfather. While still a minor, Becky reported the abuse to two LDS bishops who both informed her that *she* was forgiven and did nothing to intervene or report the crime. When a junior high school Spanish teacher, an active Mormon priesthood holder, returned missionary and married father of three, sexually abused her, Becky thought it best to tell no one. She grew up in Roy, Utah.

Rena, Janelle, Jenny and Kari
Case 04, Three Generations: More than 50 years of abuse of girls and women in the same family raped and molested by 3Ms. Fourteen-year-old Rena, the daughter of lifelong Mormons, is given over to marry an older man because his parents are "front-row members" of the church. They have four children.

Rena's second oldest daughter Janelle, as a toddler, was abused by this father, who later served time for statutory rape of his second wife's daughters. He spent 5 years in prison.

Janelle married in her teens and had a daughter, Jenny, who was sexually abused by her Mormon stepfather beginning when she was 10 years old. This man, who had three children with the victim's mother, was prosecuted and served only 3 months in jail. After his divorce from Jenny's mother, the pedophile married another women in the LDS temple and started a new family. Janelle's second daughter, Kari, was molested by "Officer Friendly," a Layton policeman who sexually abused children for seven more years before being prosecuted.

Rena is in her 60s, Janelle is 49, Jenny is 31 and Kari is 20. They grew up in Roy and Layton, Utah.

Sheri, Case 05
No Safe Haven: A 46-year-old biracial woman who has been fully raped for as long as she can recall in the home of her great-aunt and uncle, a white Mormon. To escape, Sheri married at 16. Her older husband ended up raping then having two children with her 15-year-old daughter. Sheri grew up in Salt Lake City.

Kirk, Case 06
Grandma's Favorite: A 14-year-old residential treatment client who suffers from depression. This white Mormon from Salt Lake Valley tells the shocking story of molestation and rape from the time of his earliest memories by his LDS grandmother. Kirk thought this normal as it's all he's ever known. Though therapists know of the incest, Kirk is allowed to visit his grandmother.

Annette, Case 07
Family Affairs: A 19-year-old white female with a long history of rape by her mother and father, a "stake" president (a Mormon priesthood holder over several congregations called "wards"). Annette tells of family group sex, and regular sexual assaults by her brothers, the last time "for good luck" right before one of them left for his LDS mission. She's from Salt Lake City.

Linda, Case 08
Polygamy's Daughter: A 34-year-old white single mother of four, Linda was 6 years old when her three teenage brothers tied her to the bed and raped her. The assaults lasted two years. They raped two other sisters and sodomized three brothers. The 7th of 11 children, Linda is the daughter of a Mormon polygamist who had five wives and 36 children. She's from Murray, Utah.

Crystal, Case 09
Ritualized Abuse: This 37-year-old white female, mother of six, was ritually abused by LDS priesthood holders from the time she was a baby. The Mormon wife left her husband and five children when she started to experience personality disorders associated with childhood rape and incest. She has since sought therapy and is raising a toddler son by another partner. Crystal grew up in Arizona and Utah.

36

Daddy's Girl

Awakened again by that smell, that disgusting odor that always means he's going to do it again, . . . I clench my fist, slowly tightening my body into a knot and praying it is only a dream . . . a nasty nightmare that I will soon leave in the world of dreams, once I wake. Once I wake.

My father stands over me. Fear twists my belly like every time before. Please, somebody call him away. Come to the door, ring the phone, stop him! It always takes forever. Where is Mom? Where are my brothers? How come no one ever comes in to stop him? We all fear him. I do as I'm told.

Janet grew up in the Mormon church under the control of her father. The eldest child, she has three brothers. "My earliest memories of my relationship with my father was that it was not a normal one, but I knew nothing else," she says.

Her father was "loud, large and in charge," intimidating and controlling his wife and children using any means necessary. He exercised his authority with physical beatings, emotional abuse, name calling and character assassination.

Janet's mother is submissive and afraid. She too has been raped, sodomized and beaten more times than she can count.

"When my dad beat me, mom would watch and step in only when I was bleeding too much," Janet says. "Or when I was on the floor unconscious, she would say, *Stop It, Jack, she's had enough!* Why didn't she protect me?"

Rape In The Mountains

"The sexual part started with him trying to look at my privates and touch me. I was about 14," Janet says. "Then he took me up into the mountains and made me to give him a blow job until he came in my mouth. I screamed, spit it out and felt sick. On the way home, all he did was curse me out. He said if I told anybody, he would kill me and bury me over the hill."

In 1979, Janet told a girlfriend about the abuse. "My friend was shocked but she understood because she was molested by her stepfather, too. She told her mom," Janet says. "Her mom reported it, but nothing happened because my dad hadn't had intercourse with me at that point."

Interviewing Janet is very difficult for me and her frequent tears are often joined by my own.

"Aside from beating the living shit out of me all the time, my dad was always trying to have sex with me," Janet says. "He succeeded when I was 18 after I had sex with a boyfriend. He said, *If you can fuck someone else, you can fuck me."*

Her father made three to four other children with other women while married to Janet's mother. Janet's half-sister also has been raped by this 3M for years.

"I often wondered where mom was when dad was raping me. How could she *not* know? Why didn't she stop him?" Janet sighs and starts to cry again. "He was getting into bed with me. Taking me into the mountains. Jacking off on me when I wouldn't suck him. He would hold me down and rape me in my bed while my mother was at work. The first time he raped me outside in the mountains. Then he took me to an abandoned house and raped me there."

When Janet's father didn't threaten to kill her, he bribed her to stay silent. *"If you keep your mouth shut, I'll give you a convertible Chrysler Lebaron for your very own,"* he told me.

"I wore a mask in high school because I was being hurt so bad at home," Janet says. "I was a checker at the grocery store and dad would beat me before work. He would beat me when I had trouble with math. I was very loud or very soft. I stuffed my feelings and put on this clown face like I was always happy. When I was 22, I started suffering from deep depression."

Even after getting married and moving from the house, Janet did not find peace. "Dad took me and my newborn son to Wyoming to rape me again," she says. "First, he hit me on the way there to soften me up. I was 25 years old, still nursing my son. Dad wanted me to calculate the mileage and I didn't do it right so he back-handed me in the face. Blackened my eyes, busted my nose and busted my lips with one blow. *Shut the fuck up, you're alright*, he said."

After her dad raped her in Wyoming, Janet reported the sexual assault to police there. Law enforcement there still has a completed rape kit in evidence. The state refused to prosecute and wanted no part of what appeared to be a grown woman's incest case against her father.

38

Janet also declined to prosecute. She does use the existence of the evidence and report as leverage against her father when she feels brave.

It's Done, Get Over It

Janet says she didn't resist the rapes after the age of 30: "I just let him do it without a fight or complaining too much."

I ask her if she ever initiated sex with her father.

"No. Never," she says. "I just stopped resisting and let him do it to get it over with."

Today, Janet's mother says the same thing she said from the time the Wyoming police became involved. *"Don't put your dad in jail. It's over now. Just move on with your life.* That's how my mother feels, like I can just put it behind me," she says.

Child sexual abuse and rape are not like tonsillitis. The victim cannot just "get over it." Without professional help, the psychological, emotional, and behavioral scars prohibit the person from living a healthy adult life.

First, molested adults must heal the wounds of the past. That takes a consistent personal and professionally guided effort. The wounded adult must adopt better tools to cope. The victim must change self-defeating, self-destructive behaviors and often must seek treatment for mental illness that may include severe depression, suicidal thoughts and suicide attempts, bi-polar disorder, anxiety and panic attacks.

Victims may also fall prey to drug addiction (prescription and illicit drugs) or suffer from eating disorders such as chronic overeating, anorexic nervosa or self-starvation, and the binge-and-purge cycle of bulimia. Some even resort to self-mutilation to deal with psychological turmoil. Unless victims seek and get adequate professional help, they will continue to make poor choices in life that put themselves and their children at great risk for further victimization.

Second, sexual predators need to be punished! Would Janet's mother tell her to drop the case if a stranger raped her and beat her? If parents and other relatives know they can rape and molest children without consequence, they will continue to do so.

Janet is 39 years old. She has been raped by her father for 25 years.

The Cycle Continues

Janet says that in 1984 she married a man much like her father in his abusive nature and need for absolute control. She says of her ex-husband: "I married the wrong guy, he wanted to fuck me while he wore ladies panties or women's high heels. He walked around the house in women's clothes . . . He'd punch me and kick me very hard in the vagina. He put me down verbally every day of our married life."

After her divorce, Janet says she had "the most normal relationship I'd had in years with a black man I was dating. My mom asked me if dad raped me while I was with my boyfriend. He didn't then. Once we broke up, dad came back around and depression set in again. I wanted to die."

Janet admits, "When I got suicidal, I would keep my son home with me from school so that I wouldn't kill myself."

Her ex-husband, also a Utah Mormon, has a history of child male molestation, homosexuality and cross-dressing. During one of our several interviews, Janet becomes teary eyed when seeing a male who appears to be a cross dresser. The bisexual father, now remarried with a 4-year-old daughter, was propositioned by his LDS mother several times when he was a teen.

Just a month ago, this man won legal custody of the couple's 15-year-old son after the boy spent time in an adolescent psychiatric facility under suicide precautions. Previously, the father hadn't seen his son for eight years though they live in the same area. "I'm just so scared for my son," Janet says. "I miss him and he wants to come home."

Janet's son is fully aware that his grandfather regularly rapes his mom. In fact, he was often present or within earshot of the incestual rape in progress throughout most of his life. On one occasion, her son told his grandfather: *"I hate you for what you did to my mom. You're a sick person. You need help!"*

Social services contacted Janet's ex-husband regarding their son's placement in day treatment for psychiatric problems including suicidal ideation, depression and possible bi-polar disorder. The son had violently attacked his mother and hit her several times before she literally knocked him off her. She had him emergency admitted to the local psychiatric hospital.

40

Living Without Boundaries

Before the custody hearing, Janet and her son's father started talking on the phone for hours and spending time in private at her apartment. She admits to having unprotected sex with him. She knows better. All her life she has had a difficult time setting boundaries for herself and others even when it endangers her life and the safety of her son.

During this most recent sexual relationship, her ex-husband wore pumps and women's clothing while having her perform oral sex on him. She has photographs of him in drag.

"He came over all excited and said, *Stay here, I want to show you something.* He came back dressed in a wig, my favorite dress and pumps," she says.

This new fling only lasted long enough for the ex-husband to gather information to use against Janet in the custody hearing. Janet went unprepared to the hearing and did not present the evidence she had of her ex-husband's sexual history and recent actions. My social observations of Janet reveal poor boundary setting and a strong lack of street sense. She is too trusting of strangers, lacks self-esteem, and is loud and vulgar in public. She is 5 feet, 8 inches tall and weighs 250 pounds.

Janet, who says she is not bisexual, has engaged in frequent random sexual encounters. She now dates a bisexual man whom she says she "stole" from her best girlfriend. She spends many of her days and nights at the residence of her bisexual boyfriend who lives with his dominant mother.

"He is sensitive, kind and treats me with respect," she says of her new boyfriend. "I need that in my life. He's 27 years old. But that doesn't matter, I believe he really cares for me." I ask Janet: Do you think that he only likes women now?

"I don't know."

Does he act heterosexual since being with you?

"Well, one day when I was going down on him, he said, Hey, I'm jealous because you are having all the fun! *Another time, he masturbated in front of me and ate his own semen," Janet says. "That just blew me away. I didn't know what to say."*

Does he have a history of being raped and molested?

"I think his father did it to him as a child. When I saw them together, they didn't get along at all.

"His father has issues with him being with a female. When we met, his dad asked my boyfriend, So who is this supposed to be . . . your girlfriend? I thought you're supposed to be gay!"

Have you introduced your son to your bisexual boyfriend?

"No, not yet."

Can you trust this boyfriend, a man who said he craves oral sex with other men, around your son?

"I think so."

Still Wanting A Father

Janet's feelings for her parents vacillate widely from hate and disgust to love and loyalty. "Mom was a good parent when she didn't have her blinders on," she says. "And my dad was a good father, I mean he taught me a lot, when he wasn't raping or molesting me."

Janet, who enjoys singing country music, says that she recently taped a song and dedicated it to her dad. She said he cried when he heard it. With all he's done to her, she still seeks his approval and values his opinion. She knows Dad will rape her again when given the opportunity because he has every time before. "He called me early in the morning the other day," she says, "and was masturbating to the sound of my voice."

"I'm sick and tired of being afraid of my dad! I was so tired one day and my dad found out where I lived. I woke up with him standing over me, he broke in through the window, pulled his penis out, made me suck it then he raped me. Mom was out on the front porch. He told her to wait outside."

Janet regularly talks with her parents over the phone, laughs and chats as if in an average healthy relationship. I was present on one such occasion and I witnessed classic clinical victim mentality during this dynamic. When she is apart from her father's influence, Janet exerts her independence by condemning his actions. "He put me in the role of his wife, his lover, instead of the role of daughter," she says shouting. "He robbed me of my independence and my life!"

When he comes into her space, Janet once again becomes the submissive child victim. She splits from being aware and empowered to being intimidated and submissive. The control he has over her is long standing and powerful still.

Ten minutes earlier she had been crying about her father and the years of rape and molestation, calling him a monster for ruining her life. Then he calls. They carry on a long jovial conversation It seems almost like a talk with a friend. That "friend" raped her in her home just months earlier. They laugh and curse, talking for about 30 minutes. Janet does seem tense and anxious, talking with wide volume variation, somewhat on edge, cursing occasionally in accordance with the topic of the moment.

She became tearful and confused afterward. "After raping me, dad would be silent. When he did say something he would be harsh, short winded and vulgar," she says. "I know my dad loves me and I love him, too. But he's this monster!"

This fall, Janet invited her parents to hear her sing. I also attended and met them. Her mother appeared to be quiet and submissive. When introduced to me, her father made limited eye contact, gave a brief handshake, said nothing and looked away. From my experience and further inquiry, it was apparent that the molester is also racist. All three, father, mother and Janet, are morbidly obese, ranging from 200 to 300 pounds. I suspect the family uses food and obsessive overeating to suppress uncomfortable emotions.

Raised oriented to the Christmas traditions, Janet has not returned this writer's calls during the holidays. A little investigation reveals that in order to secure Christmas money to buy presents for her son, family members and friends, Janet went to her father. Dear-old dad took full advantage of his daughter's vulnerability. He raped her and coerced her into oral sex with him in exchange for money to purchase gifts. With an income of less than $300 a month while on social security disability, Janet had been living in a Section 8 rent-subsidized apartment. Just last month, January 2002, Janet moved quite close to her childhood home.

As soon as she had her son for the weekend, she took him straight away to her parent's house for a visit.

43

Perverted Parents

She is supposed to be reading "Green Eggs and Ham" or maybe talking with her stuffed animals until she drifts off to sleep. Three-year-old Deon doesn't know that. All she knows is that this is all she's ever known — she's once again naked in bed with her mother and father, having sex.

"As far back as I can remember I was in my mom and dad's bed. We were all naked and they had me right in the middle of their sex act. They were orally and manually having sex with me, too," says the 26-year-old mother of two. "After I got older I just thought that this behavior was normal until I was allowed to visit other families. That's when I knew that what we did was not normal." Deon, who grew up in the LDS church, says that by the time she was about 13 years old, she was "used to it."

Did you and your parents ever talk about what you were doing?
>*"Yeah. They both said, What happens in this house, stays in this house," she says, "It was our little white secret."*

Did you ever have boyfriends?
>*"Not for a long time. They kept boys away from me and I was not allowed out of the house much at all."*

As you grew up, did you try to avoid sex with your parents?
>*"Yes! That's when they started getting me drunk, and then they would rape me!"*

Both of them?
>*"Yes, my mom and my dad. They would make me take off all of my clothes and take a bath, then they would come in and start molesting me in the bathroom. From there, they'd go to the bedroom or any other room in the house."*

Do you have children of your own?
>*"Yes, I have a 4-year-old little girl."*

Do you still live with your parents?
>*"Yes, well . . ., I just don't know what to do!"*

Do you think that your parents are doing to your little girl what they've been doing to you for more than 20 years?
>*"Yeah, they are! At first they would volunteer to keep her and tell me to take a break or spend the night with friends."*

During those breaks, Deon would sometimes participate in prostitution. She would sell herself for five or ten dollars, just enough to buy any drug, from whiskey to heroine, that might take her pain away and make her forget for a little while.

"My parents would push the issue, asking me to leave, until I would go for a few days. That's how it started."

What do you mean?

"Ummmm, well, now we're all in bed together!"

What are you saying? Are they now molesting your daughter, too, with you present?

"Yeah. That's what they're doing!" Deon says crying.

How often do you leave your baby girl with your parents?

"Mostly a couple of times per week. A few days at a time."

Why do you allow this molestation and rape to continue?

"My parents don't want me to work because I have to watch my little girl during the day."

Why don't you seek some assistance and just move away?

"I, I don't know, I'm, I'm scared . . . I need help . . . I'm depressed . . . I have trouble getting started, motivated."

This victim's weight has almost doubled since I first met her 18 months ago. She is now close to 300 pounds. She has openly expressed being very depressed and on medication, like so many women in Utah.

Drugs Won't Do It

In a state basically run by a religious group, it is worth mentioning that more women in Utah take mood- and mind-altering prescription drugs than in most other states. More than 90% of the women I have met and talked with here are taking prescription medication now or have been in the past.

There was a woman I met, 40 years old, beautiful, talented, from a wealthy Mormon family, a former ballroom dance champion who could sing her butt off. Emotionally, though, she was a child.

Her ex-husband, an active Mormon, had custody of her five children. Prior to physically separating from her husband, he would keep her over medicated on the wrong drugs locked inside their bedroom when he was home from work. She recalls hearing her children on the other side of the door, 'Daddy can mommy come out? We want to see mommy."

While she was drugged and naked, he would come in and rape her repeatedly, always making sure she took her medication. Her husband expected her to be gorgeous, perfectly coifed, and thin to the point of anorexia. (Her father bought her fake breasts.) She divorced and remarried this man four times.

After she separated from him, I had the opportunity to spend some time with her. I advised her to get a new psychiatric evaluation. The doctor discovered she was on the wrong medicine, tranquilizers that her husband had been feeding her, and put her on Lithium to control her manic-depression. Before her medication was adjusted, I witnessed my first manic episode one-on-one with this woman in her home. It lasted three days.

One moment she was crying, the next she would laugh uncontrollably, holding her stomach and rolling on the floor. We would listen to the radio and sing happily together. Then a song would come on that reminded her of her four boys and she was reduced to tears. That day seemed to last forever. During this period, she ran out of the house, barely dressed. Always concerned with her looks, she had to be sexy to anyone and everyone which meant she had very few personal boundaries. Before I realized she was having a manic episode, she had gone to the mailbox, and right away she met a man, he had her in his apartment, giving her a massage, had most of her clothes off, then she remembered something I had told her about predators and escaped before he could force sex.

One night she came to a club to watch me sing. She wouldn't come in. When I went outside, I saw that she had makeup bottles lined up all along the railing. When she saw me, she ran down 10 steps and hid under them. "I don't want you to see me, my makeup's not on yet!" That's when I realized just how ill she was. She was admitted to the psychiatric ward a few days later. After she was released, she left Utah with her parents who thanked me for getting her some help.

Medicated Victims

So let's look at this. Many Utah women are on mind- and mood-altering medications and are having more babies than *any other state in the country*. (I guess if molesters keep the moms medicated, they have better access to all these poor babies.)

46

And Utah has one of the highest rape/molestation rates in the country. Thus, as adults many of these victims are now knowingly or unknowingly subjecting their children to the same fate. Some victims even become perpetrators of the same crimes done against them as children.

A lot of medications mask the problem that causes the symptoms. Getting to the other side takes going through the pain, not around it, digging it all up, not burying it. If a victim must take medication especially for depression or anxiety then he or she should also seek professional counseling to deal with the aftermath of sexual abuse. Some find that after working through their feelings and changing self-destructive behaviors, they are able to live drug-free and pain-free lives.

Predators use isolation to maintain control. Medication can be part of that control. With most, if not all of the cases studied, the victim is kept away from the public, peers, other cultures and any one or group (if sub-culturally) perpetrated as in the case with culturally tolerated rape and molestation.

Deon's parents kept their daughter away from others for most of her life. She had very limited interaction with school peers and neighbors. She is now, as an adult, still overshadowed by both parents and her interaction with others is quite limited.

Though chronologically she is nearly 30, emotionally Deon has not yet moved on to adulthood. Her parents are very much her superiors and their opinion of her and her life has value to her although they are her abusers.

I observed the interaction between Deon and her dad one day at a public park. Her father was very present when she moved about. I overheard Deon ask her dad if she could go with friends to another area of the park. Her dad flatly told her, *No!* She was 25 years old at the time.

Recent contact with Deon reveals that her first daughter's father has taken custody of her 4-year-old. Thank God! She now has a 3-month-old baby girl. I believe that Deon's dad fathered this new daughter. She opts not to say who the father is, breaking eye contact with me, after I ask the question.

This young woman's life represents a sad scenario all too typical in Utah. She is a victim conditioned from birth who reverts back to being a submissive, obedient child expecting to be abused when she is with her parents.

The only plus in her story is the fact that her first daughter is now safe with her own biological father as this story is being told. Deon appears to be depressed and lost in her dilemma. There may still be hope for her new infant daughter if she and her baby get as far away from her parents as humanly possible.

The cycle must end! Deon has yet to turn her parents in for child rape and molestation. I pray that God grants her the strength and wisdom to save her baby and break the cycle. After receiving this new information, I asked Deon to give me a call and update me on how she is doing. I have yet to hear from her.

Step Monster

That couch is always very rough, made of a heavy, dark pink embroidered material. He is naked there, holding something in his hands. My sister is ironing her clothes for school. He calls us both to the couch. We have to take off our nightgowns. He makes us touch and kiss this thing between his legs.

"Lick it like an ice-cream cone," he says. I feel scared and bad, like I'm a bad girl. This man might be my new dad soon. He smells like beer and Old Spice. Maybe this is what dad's do. He puts his fingers between my legs. It hurts. He keeps me there on that rough couch. Then he tells us to get ready and go to school. I'm in first grade.

It seems everybody liked Stan, a gregarious businessman born and raised in Utah. He was a personable salesman involved in politics and stressing the importance of a college education. Stan projected the perfect picture of a man concerned with the future of his community and his family. A harsh disciplinarian, he expected the best of himself and others.

People remember the pride Stan took in his youngest stepdaughter. Becky was intelligent, talented and attractive. An active member of the Mormon church, she was also a virgin – a fact which made her stepfather very proud. Sometimes Stan would take Becky on visits around town just to show her off and brag about her straight A's. Valedictorian of her high school, on the marching team, her future shining ahead of her, in part, because stepdad taught her so well and cared so much.

48

Of course, those who knew him best, his wife of 10 years and his four stepchildren, knew his other side – binge drinking, violence, threats, abuse – just as law enforcement in his hometown of Ogden knew him to be a hot-tempered alcoholic. But Stan talked a good line and fooled many people into believing the enviable public picture he painted of himself.

Every Night A Nightmare

Stan began sexually abusing Becky when she was 6 years old and continued until she was 17. Her entire childhood lost to this man. He molested her two older sisters as well. In fact, Becky told her mom about the sexual abuse after the first incident. Her mother confronted Stan and he said he wouldn't do it again. He lied. From that point on it happened almost every night.

"At our first house, my two sisters and I shared a room. He would molest us one at a time while the other two remained frozen with fear. I just held my breath. I knew I was next," Becky says. "My mom had to know he wasn't in her bed. Where did she think he was?" During the day, Stan would act as though everything was normal. *"Oh, you girls are the greatest kids!"* he'd say. "He'd take us places, snowmobiling, drive-in movies, buy us things."

Becky remembers one incident that really messed with her head. She was 9 years old.

"We all went to a drive-in movie in the car. It seems Stan and I were in the back seat. That's weird, don't you think, us in the back seat, mom in the front. Or maybe I just wished we were in the back seat so I could pretend she (mom) didn't know what was going on. We were watching *Straw Dogs* with Dustin Hoffman, rated R. It showed a woman getting raped, full frontal nudity. Mom and Stan are talking about how they didn't know it was rated R or they wouldn't have brought us.

"Stan pushes my head down against the seat so I can't see the atrocities on the screen and all the while he has his fingers under my panties in my vagina!"

As Becky and her sisters came home from school when her mom was still at work, Stan would push one or the other of them into a corner and force himself on her. *"Gotta see how you're growing,"* he'd say to Becky, shoving his one hand under her training bra and the other into her underwear.

Even when their mother *was* home, Stan would pinch all three girls on the buttocks, come up behind them and put his hands on their breasts while they did the dishes. He would have Becky stay up and watch *Nightmare* on television with him every week. While he lay on the couch totally naked, he had Becky lie in front of him concealing his demented acts with a blanket, strip her and finger rape her for the entire program.

Then one night Becky thought she was going to die. She was about 11 years old. "I was in my room sleeping and heard my older sister crying from her bedroom across the hall, *Please don't do this to me. I don't want to. Just leave me alone.*

"My whole body was shaking and I could barely walk I was so scared but I made it into the hall. I screamed: Leave My Sister Alone! He was out of the room in a flash, grabbed me by the neck and pulled my whole body up by my head.

"He slammed me against the wall almost to the ceiling. I couldn't breathe. His face was red, his eyes unnatural: *Don't tell me what to do or I will kill you!* I was blacking out. I thought he was going to snap my neck. Then, he let go. I collapsed."

After she told her mom about being choked, Becky remembers getting a break from Stan's nightly perversions when her mother and stepdad separated. As soon as they decided to reconcile, a very disturbing incident occurred.

"One day my mom took me to Stan's apartment in Salt Lake City for a visit," Becky says. "After we greeted him, I don't know where mom went. Now I'm in the shower with my stepdad and we are both totally naked. (Like this is normal behavior?) I was probably 12 at the time.

"Did mom go to the store or what? Was she waiting in the living room? Where was she actually? How could she not know? Was she just doing what she was told, was she afraid, was she looking for a weapon, was she gathering courage or was she reading a magazine? Whatever she was doing, she was not there to protect me *again*.

"I remember being in the shower and him rubbing soap all over my body. Then I remember him sticking his penis in my face. That's all I remember to this day. I don't remember the rest of the shower, getting out or even going home . . . Even if my mom wasn't there, she had to have noticed my wet hair. She asked me no questions. It wasn't a source of concern at all."

50

Soon Stan was back in the home and the abuse continued into her teens. When she was 16, Becky told a Mormon bishop about the 10 years of abuse. He told her, *"God will forgive you, you can be certain of that."* The comment made Becky feel like the abuse was her fault.

They Turned A Deaf Ear

"When I was 16 I had an interview with my bishop to attain a temple recommend so I could get baptized for the dead," Becky says. "I had to confess any sin that I thought might keep me from the temple, especially any moral or sexual sin to a man who was obviously not experienced as a counselor.

"I always thought the abuse was partly my fault. Maybe I was too close to Stan. Maybe I just let it happen because he would pay attention to me and give me gifts and treat me better than my sisters and brother. So I told my bishop that my stepfather was touching my body." Becky's bishop was silent. "His face went really red. Then after awhile he said, *Well, I really don't know what we can do about that. Have you ever initiated this type of activity with him?* I told him no that he does it mostly when he is drunk at night and comes into my bedroom. I just pretend to be asleep.

"'I want you to know,' the bishop said, 'that <u>you</u> are forgiven for your part in this.' Then the bishop told me how careful I must be not to find myself alone with adult males or peers," Becky says. "I remember this well because it made me feel ashamed and uncomfortable." The bishop continued: '*You are a very attractive young lady. If you dress provocatively or give young men any reason to believe you are easy, they will take advantage of you. Watch how you dress, how you act and who you are with. Do not get into petting or kissing. Do not let anyone touch you under your clothes. Okay?'*

"Then he gave me my temple recommend. I had worn what I thought was a conservative dress to the interview, a straight Army-type olive green dress with buttons down the front. I asked the bishop if this was an appropriate dress. He said it was not. I developed early and I guess the dress showed my curves," Becky says. "While I was walking home from the church a group of guys whistled at me and yelled at me to join them in the truck. I ran into my grandma's house nearby and just cried hysterically.

51

"The bishop was right. It is my fault. I make these men act this way. I'm a slut. I must give off some kind of nasty vibe. What can I do to stop this from happening?"

Becky told another bishop about Stan's criminal acts a year later and he too said, *"Be assured that you are forgiven. God will take care of your stepfather."* No one reported this serial child rapist to police.

Fed To The Wolf

The molestation usually took place at night, until Becky turned 17 years old then Stan sexually abused her in the daytime, twice. The first of these occurred in the bathtub.

"He told me I had to shave the pubic hair from inside my thighs so I could wear my swimsuit. *I'll do it for you*, he said. I was naked in the tub and he began shaving me, one hand with the razor and the other probing between the lips of my vagina," Becky says. "For the first time in my life, I could see what he was doing. And suddenly I realized my throat was tight, my breath quick. I was getting turned on and it scared the hell out of me! I grabbed the razor and told him to leave. He said no and protested. I stood up naked in the tub and just yelled at him, "Get out!"

One day soon thereafter, Becky's mom was out of town traveling with her job, and Stan was out of work, drunk and home alone with his stepdaughter.

"I was cleaning my bedroom and Stan called me from his room," Becky says. "I opened the door to his room. He was masturbating on his waterbed. He said, *Come here. Take it.* It was weird. I could have walked away. It was like I was 6 years old again. I sat on the bed. He put both my hands around his penis and made me move it up and down. He tried to put his fingers in my white shorts. I said, No! He said, *I need to. It helps.* He shoved his fingers inside me then ejaculated all over my hands."

Becky went into Stan's bathroom and washed her hands with a foot brush, scrubbing them until they were red and raw. When she came out, she said, "I will never do that again."

"I had to say something because I had this overwhelming feeling that I was going to go to hell for doing what I did for him and allowing him to touch me."

Stan replied, *"You must really love me to do that for me when you didn't want to."*

52

"I was disgusted, physically ill really, and just fed up. I was packing a suitcase to run away to my best friend's house when my brother interrupted me. I was embarrassed. I couldn't tell him what happened. I said I was upset about Stan's drinking."

Her brother had just returned from a Mormon mission and he did what they were all taught to do. "Let's pray," he said.

"That just shut me down. I was too ashamed to say anything after that," Becky says.

She did tell her mom though. At that time, Becky didn't have any conscious memory of ever telling her mother about the abuse. When she revealed the most recent incident. her mom said, *"Oh, you girls told me that when you were little."*

(Author's Note: If mom had acted when she first heard the news when Becky was 6 years old she could have stopped a decade of abuse perpetrated against three little girls.)

Soon Becky was off to college and her mom started divorce proceedings to break once and for all from Stan.

Stan continued to harass Becky by phone when she was attending college in Logan. "He called and asked if I was a virgin. He said, *Well, I'm not your real father so we can have sex. It wouldn't be incest.* I was appalled. I didn't know what to say. I gave him some psycho-babble about needing a parental figure not a lover. Then he said, *It wasn't that bad. What I did to you girls wasn't that bad."*

He called again when Becky was 22 years old and working as a reporter at a daily newspaper. "He wanted me to come to Ogden and visit him before he moved away with his new wife. First, though he asked how much I weighed. *I don't want to be seen with a fat girl,* he laughed. He had planted the seed of thin in all of us, in me and my sisters. We had to be thin to be valued. My oldest sister was bulimic and I was a chronic overeater who would have blackout eating sessions where I'd down a whole bag of chips in one sitting and not remember doing it.

"Stan constantly told me and my sisters. *You will never get a husband, never have children, never land a job, if you are fat.* I weighed 125 pounds in high school. Anorexia was rampant in my school. So, of course, I thought I was huge. I was not fat."

"The whole conversation, he was so pathetic. I hung up on him," Becky says. That was the last time she talked to Stan. He now lives in Louisiana with his wife and her grown children.

"I pity that family. I worry for any grandchildren that might come to visit him," Becky says. "A pedophile never changes unless maybe he is forced to by getting caught and locked up. *Stan doesn't even think he did anything wrong!* I think he feels like it was his right. He has this sick sexual need and kids exist in his life to fulfill it."

Some Are Called Teachers

With so many issues at home, Becky became quite involved in school activities. She was voted president of the Spanish club at age 13. "One day my Spanish teacher invited me and another girl, the vice president, to a club planning meeting. I was leery because he had already touched me once," Becky says.

"I was staying after school to take a make-up test and he came up behind me to see how I was doing. He pointed to something on the paper then placed his hand on my breast. *You have the most beautiful breasts in this whole school. I can't believe it, you're becoming a woman.* I shrugged and told him I had to finish and get home. I didn't know what to say. I just shut my mouth like I did at home every night."

The meeting took place at the other girl's neighborhood where there was a swimming pool. "So we went to my friend's house and it was apparent this man did not want to have a Spanish Club meeting. He brought an older friend, a Mexican native who was also Mormon. They talked about his recent conversion. Then we all went swimming. My teacher came up behind me and put his hand in my bikini bottoms. Donna was across the pool with the other man and I just assumed he was doing the same to her. Neither one of us ever talked about it.

"After I left junior high school I received a valentine from my old Spanish teacher that said on the front, *I Can't Wait To Get My Hands On You!* I didn't tell my mom or stepdad because I knew it wouldn't matter. He wrote a bunch of stuff inside the card in Spanish and since I never learned Spanish, although he gave me straight A's, I have no idea what it said."

It didn't end there. "My senior year in high school, the Spanish teacher called me up and asked me if he could see me before he moved to Jackson County, Missouri. He was an active Mormon and believed the saints would eventually gather there for the second coming of Jesus Christ.

"We rode around in his car talking about school and stuff then he asked me to come with him. *I want you to come with me and my family. I want you to be my second wife.* I was shocked and a little frightened. I asked him to take me home. We drove up into my driveway and parked. He asked for a hug. I gave him one. He pulled me into him and gave me a fumbling open-mouthed kiss. I was shaking, backed out of the car and slammed the door. I never told anyone about him until today." As far as she knows, this man is teaching in Missouri.

Healing The Wounds

After her first serious panic attack in 1993, Becky had to face the demons of her past. "I knew I was going crazy. I'd just begun a new job, filed for bankruptcy, separated from my husband, lost my grandmother to a rest home, and, at 30 years old, moved back home with my mother," Becky says. "I was seriously depressed – endlessly watching television, digging at my toenails, biting my fingernails, burying myself in 30 extra pounds – for a whole year.

"I cried uncontrollably to my sister over the phone, then afterward picked up a newspaper to try and relax. When I read the word *schizophrenic* in a news story, it was like a gigantic gray egg cracked over my head – my vision clouded, my heart raced, I ran outside to catch my breath. The world contracted in on me. I thought the sky was about to crash down. I ran. It took four hours of walking the neighborhood that I did not recognize as my own, to finally feel somewhat normal. I made it home when I spent all my energy and calmed down. But I knew something was terribly wrong. Ironically, a few days later, as a writer in university public relations, I covered a meeting about incest survivors on campus. The counselor described a panic attack! She said the disorder afflicts adults molested or raped as children. I had a name and a reason for my crazy experience, my nervous breakdown.

"After 10 phone calls talking with people who told me I needed insurance, two months on a waiting list or a discounted fee of $85 per session for therapy, I finally got an understanding and knowledgeable social worker on the phone who was facilitating free group therapy for adults molested as children. A shaking shell of a person, I was sure my therapist would have to put mental hospital for life and I told her I thought she should. She said there were other things I could do to heal.

55

"She gave me a listening ear, asked important questions and provided me with coping skills. In group therapy, I learned that some of the clichés I heard from self-help books had some real power behind them:

You've Got To Feel To Heal
I must go through the pain not around it.
Talk about what happened, don't ignore it.
Talk with and/or confront the people involved.

Go Ahead and Get Angry
Make a commitment to no longer hurt myself or those I love.
Yell at my perpetrator, not my partner.
Shame my abuser, not myself.

Listen To The Child Inside
Call her *sweetheart* instead of *stupid*.
Nurture yourself; be the kind of mother you never had.
When feelings confuse me, ask her what she is trying to say.

Tell The Secret
Share the horror with someone who will understand.
Take the power away from my abuser and give it to myself.
Tame the nightmares, write them down.

The Confrontation Letter
Talking with women who had similar childhoods, Becky was able to recall specific memories of abuse, write them down and finally begin to tackle her problems. One of her most important steps toward healing was to confront her stepfather with the truth that he always insisted she hide. Since she could not safely confront him in person, she wrote a detailed letter to Stan. Becky tracked down his address in Louisiana and mailed the letter to him.

"STAN – Ten years ago over the phone you said we should have sex. After all, you said, I was an adult, "no longer a virgin and we weren't related by blood." I was stunned and appalled. What you said next horrified me – *It wasn't that bad. What I did to you girls wasn't that bad.* I stopped talking to you 10 years ago but those words still echo in my head.

56

"You really don't know what happens to little girls whose stepfathers sexually abuse them, do you? You think, *It wasn't that bad. I just touched her. I told her I loved her. She was my special princess. I gave her presents. I paid attention to her. This was our little secret.* The truth is – the reality is – you invaded me! You RAPED me! How do you rape a 6-year-old? Slam your penis into her and you'll tear her up, your plaything will be destroyed and you'll get arrested. No, you rape a 6-year-old with your finger and your tongue and by shoving your penis in her mouth. You took my body over as your toy. I was a baby. A child. I wanted to be loved. I wanted a dad. I was tiny, trusting and vulnerable. Frightened. Scared shitless. And you continued your selfish perversions for more than 10 years.

"My entire childhood. I knew nothing else. What a bastard. Okay, here, I'll give it to you straight so you can't sugarcoat it with any of your fatherly-love bullshit. You shoved your penis into my hands, my face, my mouth when I was too young to comprehend what the thing even was. You shoved your fingers into my vagina. It hurt, damn it! You took my virginity. Broke my hymen. You butchered my innocence, you stripped me of my privacy and you stole what were supposed to be the most carefree days of my life.

"Then, you burglarized me every night. First, you came into my room and to my bed saying you loved me. And you hurt me. You pawed at my little girl body. You took MY body away from ME and made it yours. I felt pain. I felt fear. I felt confused. And emotionally I couldn't understand why you were so needy and cruel. Why would you hurt me? What did I do wrong?

"Then, you put your mouth on me. How is a child supposed to understand that act? The oral sex made me feel dirty and bad. I felt ashamed. Like I was a bad person. You forced me to kiss you like a lover. The memory of it nauseates me.

"So, what happens to little girls who must live with this invasion, the ones who survive the torment? The ones who don't just kill themselves to stop the pain? They have night terrors when they are 31 years old! Some disappear into the woodwork like my quiet sister and some lash out in anger like my oldest sister. Some space out like me, covering everything up with a smile and endless achievements in an attempt to prove to myself and others that nothing was amiss.

"We were real find for you, weren't we? An incest smorgasbord and you were an insatiable PIG. We weren't the only ones were we? There were others, too. Your own blood daughters. You propositioned one of them when she was pregnant, for God's sake! What kind of loser are you?

"As for me, when you ripped into my body – you tore the fabric of my mind. You set the stage for my messed up adult life. You branded me, priming me for abusive relationships, self hate, chronic overeating, drug abuse, physical disability and mental instability. You did this to me. This is your legacy as a father.

"Some of my nightmares are real. Like that night I heard my sister pleading and I screamed LEAVE HER ALONE! In the middle of the dark hall, my legs and hands shaking, *Leave my sister alone!* You bounded from her room. You grabbed me by the throat. I was 12 or 13 years old. You wrenched my head from my shoulders and slammed it against the wall and ceiling. Pinning me up there like a human noose. You said, *Don't ever tell me what to do again or I will kill you.*

"For one small moment, I spoke – I screamed – your ugly secret and you felt threatened enough to nearly take my life. What a coward you are. The memory of that night used to paralyze me. That night I learned to hate and I learned to fear. I hated and feared you. I grew to hate myself and fear life and love. I suspect anyone now who shows me even genuine affection. I figure it will end and they will hurt me. Or that they only want something for themselves.

"You taught me how demented a human can be. Intimacy is foreign to me. I have flashbacks of your hands backing me into a corner, pawing and pinching my breasts, my bottom, shoving your hands down my pants. The fear freezes me. I lash out at those I love. I have panic attacks. Sometimes, I think I'm losing my mind.

"But, you see, it's not my fault. This hideous truth is on your shoulders. Yes, I must deal with the fallout now or die. I must take painful, positive steps to heal. The shame and guilt are yours. The courts have a name for what you did to me – *aggravated sexual abuse, a first-degree felony.* What you did is against the law, asshole! It wasn't that bad, you say? Men like you, who prey on children, can spend 15 years to the rest of their lives in prison. Maybe one day you'll get elected to serve your time. Most, like you, don't spend one day in jail.

58

"What you did to me, I call it torture. Physical, emotional, psychological torture. Your punishment? To live out the rest of your life as a pathetic old man who must wear the leprous brand of CHILD MOLESTER and PEDOPHILE until the day you die. To exist in your own living hell knowing the lives you have taken. You murdered the child I could have been and the person I could have become had you never attacked me.

"Women who are abused like me, our minds split from our bodies. We dissociate and space out. We are not present during a huge part of our lives. I have avoided reality and tried to escape the paralyzing fear by always fantasizing a better and different life since I was 6 years old. I've lied to myself and others even when the truth would have better served me. I have been so angry I thought I would physically, literally explode if I had to go on living one more second. I still cry. I cry. I CRY. I scream! Then sometimes I am so silent and numb, I could pass for dead.

"I've used food like a drug to silence these feelings and cushion me from a predatory world. The irony is this – your constant sharp and critical voice pounded into my head that I must be skinny and tan at all costs to be wanted, loved and successful. Had you *not* molested me for my entire childhood, I might have had a chance to befriend my own body and allow myself to have a healthy, happy physical existence. Instead, I learned so well from you to abuse, ignore and hate my body, to hide behind fat and food much like you hide behind alcohol.

"Well, you say, these are my problems. I was always a strange, emotional, overly dramatic little girl who suffers from an overactive imagination. I say – Fuck you! Fuck you like you fucked me! Why am I still afraid to go to sleep at night? Because for every night of my young life I thought you would come.

"You would come into my room like some possessed stranger and deceive me with your loving words and rape me. Every time we watched nightmare on Friday nights, you fingered me, kissed on me, pawed and pinched me. I fled into the shows. Now those stark images wake me in terror. It wasn't fun for me. DO YOU GET IT YET? I wasn't having a good time. *No child is a willing participant in an adult's sexual perversion.* You used my childlike trust and my need to be loved to manipulate me. You forced sexual awareness on me before my time and twisted it into an instrument of power, pain and fear.

59

"From the day you masturbated in front of me and made me touch your penis when I was a child, from that first vile day forward, there was no hope of me ever having a *normal* childhood. Behind any smile I smiled as a little girl there was your ugly secret lurking like a monster. Painful. Horrible. Sick. Terrifying. You shattered any chance as a father when you forced your sex on me. That is a grave loss to any child. I ceased to feel. I literally left my body in your hands. It was mine but you took it.

"With that, you stole my self-esteem, my trust, my grip on reality and, for a very long time, my potential for any real or lasting happiness. When I got my first brand new car on my own with my own money, that night I dreamed you smashed it to pieces with a sledge hammer. You have always been waiting around the corner of any happiness I experienced ready to pounce on me. Just like you did in those houses; always invading, controlling, criticizing, molesting, raping. And even when you weren't there physically, you were. Every night for more than 10 years, I would wait in my bed, my eyes open wide or closed to tightly they stung, fearing that I might have to run away again in my head or seek refuge in the wall or fly out the window if you came in.

"Sometimes, I'd let myself fall asleep and feel safe only to be thrust awake by your rough, probing hands and smelly, stinking breath and your pathetic behavior. Then, I knew after so many nights like that, it was NEVER safe to sleep. So, you see, your evil, invasive, selfish presence was there every night of my life from the time I was 6 years old until you finally left the house after I graduated high school.

"Then, the nightmare of you invaded my dreams and still does to this day. You say, *it wasn't that bad, get over it already, get on with your life, put it behind you, everyone goes through some shit in their childhood.* There's no magic bandage to make these wounds heal. I can't *wish* it away. I can't *will* the stark memories to disappear. I can't *think* the panic attacks away. I can no longer pretend, I can no longer stuff the overwhelming feelings of pain, anger, hate and betrayal.

"I can no longer deny that a decade or more of your alcoholism, sexual abuse and mind control had a lasting impact on me. I was affected, deeply. To get over it, I must go straight through it, for the first time in my life.

60

"From this baggage I carry, I must drag all the dirty pieces out onto the table in full light and sort through them. That honesty will take me to the edge of sanity and create havoc in my life. But I will meet your disgusting legacy straight on and I will conquer it. Because – get this, you bastard – I am not afraid of you anymore. I am no longer scared! I am no longer silent!

"I know that you'd like to think that the success I attained in my schooling is due to you. I take that from you. You can't have it. *I made those achievements.* I threw myself into my studies and my grades and work to cope with the covert, shameful reality of our home. I avoided and denied by becoming someone everyone could count on, the peacemaker, the princess, the one who would make it right, the smart one, the untouched virgin (ha!), little Miss Perfect Straight-A Student. It was a desperate, unhealthy, dysfunctional way to live. That is how *I* survived *you*. So don't pat yourself on the back for my accomplishments. I have become more than a grade on a piece of paper.

"Writing this letter to you marks a point in my life. I'm taking my life back from you, Stan. I reclaim my body and my mind as my own. You have no power over me. I kill you. I bury you. I damn you to Hell. I damn the society of preoccupied, patriarchal, sexist, evil, self-satisfaction-at-any-cost male power structure that made you into the monster you are today.

"You say you were abused as a child and that is your excuse. I don't accept that. I do not care nor do I need to know what horrors you may have endured that led you to turn your sick perversions and selfish needs onto young girls. You are an adult. You should have taken care of it, got help, locked yourself up or killed yourself before ever laying a hand on me.

"I thank God there are some men, maybe many men, who are not like you, who don't take from children for their own warped pleasure, who get help when their past haunts them, who don't lash out at women and children. And I point the finger at those who do. I defy all you bastards! I am fighting back against every single one of you. I am screaming out your dirty little secret! I am fighting for myself, for my sisters whom I love, for those men who aren't like you, for the children you hurt and continue to hurt, for the little girls and boys you will never get at so they won't have to go through the living hell you put me through.

"And I am fighting for the many women, like my mother, whom you demeaned and paralyzed to the point that they sacrificed their babies to save themselves. So, when you say it wasn't that bad – Think Again! When you say it was just innocent touching and try to wrap it up in some noble love – Give Me A Break! When you say it wasn't rape because your penis never penetrated – Read The Law! When you rationalize that we weren't related by blood so it wasn't INCEST – Get A Clue!

"What happens to girls and boys who are sexually assaulted and psychologically raped? We grow up with an enormous strength to overcome. I am a survivor. I survived you, the worst kind of predator. I will survive the healing process. I am an educated victim with an attitude. So watch your back. *All of you molesters better watch your back.* Because we are out there full of rage and getting stronger. We will have our day.

"I am also an adult. I am getting the help I need. I have a deep spirituality and faith that give me power. I have a family who wants me to get better despite the pain it might cause them. And I have friends who lift me up because they too have been victims. Unfortunately, there are too many who were terrorized by the likes of you. You monsters give men a bad name.

"I am working through the aftermath of your abuse. I am dealing with the anger and self-destructive behaviors that grew out of your sick need to possess, invade and get off sexually. That is my responsibility. One day soon I will dispose of you, Stan. I will work through all the pain and face all the memories and, finally, go on to experience life, joy and peace. To get there, I need to know that you know just how BAD it was. I want you to feel pain. I want *you* to cry. Weep, you bastard. Weep. *–BECKY Feb. 5, 1994*"

Mom, Where Were You?

"MOM: How dare you give me a lecture on my life! My addiction to prescription pills, the binge eating, the depression, the panic attacks, the failed relationships, the promiscuity, the self-hate, the health problems, the lost jobs, the continuing need for you or someone else to rescue me from my dysfunction.

It's time that you take responsibility for *your* piece of this shit pie that is my life!

Why am I, your 40-year-old daughter, such a mess? There's a concrete reason for this. Can you guess what it is? It's not a character flaw mom, it's not a lack of discipline, it's not a moral weakness, it's not because I ditched the Mormon church. The reason? Simple: *You failed to protect me when I was a tiny girl and you were all I had.*

Do you remember when you held my hand in bed and we pointed out the monster faces cast by night shadows on the ceiling? You were frightened, too. I felt responsible to comfort you even though I was a child. I'm not the mom. You are. I write this letter to tell you about the real monsters in my life and childhood. I write this letter to let go of the fantasy mother I made you out to be, the fantasy mother you pretended to be. I'm hoping to recognize and accept the real person you are. And for you to do the same for me.

I am well aware of my part in my circumstances. I turned to prescription drugs to numb the pain and panic caused by being sexually abused for a decade. I was medicated and asleep when my daughter was molested by a member of the Mormon church. I was in the bishop's office confessing my "sins" to three strangers, when this man finger raped my baby. I failed her.

I was too busy looking for a quick fix in prescribed drugs and religion that I left my child in the hands of a pedophile. I must take responsibility for my deplorable actions. I have not continued in those behaviors. I have made bold changes.

What of you, mom? You didn't leave Stan because, you said, you were afraid he would kill you then get custody of us. Use your head, that wouldn't have happened. Even if he did kill you, we would have been elsewhere, not with him. And, believe me, anyplace but there would have been a better place to be. You were afraid he would kill us all? Newsflash! I would have preferred death. I would rather have been dead than live one more second with him raping me. He had you beat down? You should have gotten up! It was your duty to protect me. I would lay down my life for my daughter. You should have at least risked the same for me.

I know you say there was no help in those days. No social support. No safe houses. No information or education about child molestation or spousal abuse. I really try to understand this. You grew up in a supportive family, didn't you?

To me, common sense, parental instinct, a sense of moral obligation should have moved you to *throw Stan out* of our house after the first time he molested my sister and I. You weren't married to him yet. Lock the door! Get a weapon! Are you trying to tell me that my real father or his father or your father or my uncles would not have killed Stan if you turned to them for help? Why didn't you? If a stranger had raped us or you, would you let him back in the house? Would you marry him just months later? What happened to you in your childhood that made you to think what Stan did to us was in any way acceptable?

I cannot believe I have felt guilty all this time for failing you! I wasn't the great success you were counting on. Your daughter just couldn't get it together. Man, what's wrong with her? As long as I turned out all right we could all pretend that the hell we went through didn't have any impact on who we would become. My sisters have suffered, too.

You say, *"Pick up your bootstraps. Forgive yourself. Get on with your life."* It's a bit more complicated than that. I'm no magician. I can't make it disappear for you. No amount of professional success, not becoming a fabulously active and deliriously happy member of the Mormon church with a safe predictable Mormon husband, none of that would or could erase the horrifying reality of more than 10 years of child sexual abuse you allowed your mate to shit-pile upon me.

Where were you, mom? Where were you when Stan wasn't in your bed but in mine or my sisters'? Where were you when he made me and my sister masturbate his penis when I was 6 years old? We told you about it then! Why did you not leave him forever that moment? Why didn't you take a baseball bat to his head? How could you be so in need of a man that you would sacrifice your own daughters to him. Were you blind, selfish or stupid? You won't talk about your past. I suspect you were a victim in some way. However, that's no excuse. You closed your eyes and sacrificed my body and soul to this man, for what? To save yourself, to save face, to make ends meet, to have a man. There is just no good reason at all. Where were you? Where were you when he nearly choked the life out of me because I tried to stop him from raping my sister? I was in the hall yelling at him to stop, not you! Where were you when he slammed my oldest sister's face into the table because she wouldn't join the ROTC?

"Where were you when he split my other sister's lip open because she resisted? Asleep again or gone to a friend's house? Where were you when he took me into the shower with him during our visit to his Salt Lake apartment? *You drove me there, mom.* Where were you when he made fun of my breasts, my thighs and my butt? You giggled with him about the buttons he sewed on the nipple parts of my training bra. You allowed us all to run around the house in our underwear in front of a grown man. How could this seem normal, healthy to you? Where were you when he scared away my boyfriends. Did you think that was a father's right or did you realize he was simply jealous of his stepdaughter's suitors? Creepy. Where were you when he forced me to masturbate him in his room when I was 17? Where were you when he shaved the inside of my legs with a razor in one hand, shoving his fingers into me with the other?

Where were you when he stole my soul and my sanity and my future and my body and my life? You were absent. You made the conscious choice to be absent.

MOTHER – WHERE THE HELL WERE YOU WHEN I NEEDED YOU TO SAVE ME FROM THIS MONSTER? Stan was not a shadow on the ceiling. He was real and you knew it. You knew more than you want to admit. I know now that you knew, that you must have known in some way all along.

You were not the mom you and I pretended you to be. Myth: You worked three jobs to take care of us. *Reality: You worked to get away from an abusive partner and left us alone to be his prey.* Myth: You were the coolest mom because you could talk to me about anything like sex or other taboos *Reality: When it came to sexual theory and the future, we talked openly. You and I ignored the present. You ignored the fact that your husband had already penetrated my vagina with his fingers, forcibly kissed me, put his penis in my mouth, dirtied and demeaned me.*

Myth: You spent extra time with me on my homework so I could be successful in school. *Reality: My schoolwork would redeem me and you. My success would prove to you and the world that this pedophile had no impact on me whatsoever. Guess what – the straight A's didn't keep the monster away.* Myth: When I told you how bad it was, you cried and asked for my forgiveness. The perfect response. *Reality: You have always known what to say, but your actions do not follow.*

65

You told me one day, "Maybe you have so many problems because you didn't have a strong father figure." Mom, I had a fucked up, mentally ill father figure. He was a criminal, a serial child molester. He raped me while you stood by and did nothing. You turned your back on me!

Even once he yelled it right out to you: *"I molested your daughters and you still want me back!"* He said that to you in a bar full of people right after you begged him to come home. You knew all along. Yes, he molested us and it did not matter to you. It did not matter. You refused to leave him or change your life. No matter how much you wanted a stable, fulfilling relationship, no matter how much you didn't want to be twice divorced, no matter how much he raped you or threatened to kill you or us – when you made a decision to bring me into this world, you took on the responsibility to protect me. You decided not to.

Do I hate you for that? I hate the part of you that sacrificed me and my sisters to save yourself. No matter how much I loved my husband, if he turned out to be a monster like Stan, I would shoot him dead and let God decide my punishment. The least I would do is leave, find help, barricade the doors, scream, stand up to him and make a decision to save my children. You did not do the least you could do. That choice forever changed my life.

Can I forgive you? You and I formed a bond when we held hands and saw monsters on the ceiling. That bond soon became a rope around my neck. Mom, I am cutting the noose. Let us be adults with each other. I don't want to lie to you anymore to make my life seem like it is what you hoped it would be.

You won't talk about your past, saying only, "Everyone goes through difficulties in childhood." Being sexually molested and psychologically battered is not a normal childhood difficulty. With that statement, I assume you have some demons of your own that you need to face head-on. The best thing you can do is talk them out with a qualified therapist. That effort would greatly improve our relationship and likely give you some peace of mind.

Nothing can erase what was done to me. I am responsible now to change my life for the better. My life choices have been based a lot on my being a victim of child sexual abuse. Now, my life choices are based on being a survivor.

Don't make me out to be a princess. Don't mark me as special, somehow apart from others. That brand only meant I had to be different, better somehow and that I could not show weakness or make mistakes. I am human. I am a woman. From one human being to another, let us be honest with each other.

Some monsters are real, mom. I will no longer pretend that Stan was a shadow on the ceiling. How you deal with that reality is your decision. May you find strength and insight to make peace with yourself. –BECKY Feb. 3, 2002"

When Becky was 31 years old, she attended a work meeting at Weber State University and sitting across from her was an old associate of Stan's. "Wow, Becky, how are you?" he said. "And how is your Dad, I haven't seen him for 10 years?"

Becky remained silent and shifted in her seat as the small group around her waited for a stereotypical kindly response. Then she looked Stan's old friend in the eye and said, "He's not my dad. He was my stepfather and he is a pedophile." Silence. Now, everyone else shifted in their seats.

"I'd just gone through 18 months of intense therapy for adults molested as children," Becky says. "I was not about to carry on the pretense just to make people feel comfortable. I think it's about time people feel uncomfortable."

Three Generations

It's my job. I will redeem our family. I will join a wealthy, respected family in the church and things will change for us. Maybe dad won't have to work so hard to make ends meet. Maybe we won't have to work so hard to fit in.

Do I love him? I don't think that matters. He's a front-row church member. I'm beautiful. I'm 14 years old. I guess it's time for me to be a wife and a mother, to have a bunch of children. That's why I'm here. That's my destiny. I might as well begin while I'm still a kid, just so I can get a good start on things.

In the late 1940s, Rena married Joe when she was 15 and he was 24. Joe was from a prominent Mormon family, they were "front-row" members, a spot for the privileged with money.

It was the tradition that poorer, less-educated beauties were offered up as prime candidates for marital servitude. Their parents wanted a piece of the economic church pie by any means even if it meant trading off of one of their own children. Imagine a young girl, immature and ignorant, whose job it was to serve her Mormon husband, with whom she had nothing in common. Joe was controlling and abusive.

Rena and Joe had their first daughter the first year of their marriage. Shortly thereafter came Janelle. This second daughter was a quiet, nervous child and a delight none-the-less. Then came a son and another daughter right in a row.

Like a majority of victims, Janelle's memories of her childhood are sketchy. She does recall one incident that would set the stage for a troubled future. "One day, I remember being in the car, I think I was with my dad," Janelle says. "Mom got out to go into some building. Dad put his hand between my legs. I was frightened. I must have been squirming because he yelled at me in this horrible voice, *Hold still!* That's all I remember."

When Janelle was 5, Joe and Rena divorced. Her dad married another woman. He started to molest and rape his new wife's daughters and nieces. She prosecuted. Joe spent five years in prison for statutory rape. "I remember he didn't feel bad about what he had done," Janelle says. "He was pissed that he'd been caught. He thought he was doing nothing wrong and nobody should interfere."

Even with Joe out of the house, Janelle still was not safe. When she was 11, she babysat for the neighbors. When they came home, and their children were asleep, before Janelle could leave, the man started touching her body through her clothes.

"He just started touching me, molesting me while his wife sat on the living room couch and watched. I kept saying I have to go home now, after saying this over and over, they finally let me leave and go home. I didn't tell my mom or my stepdad. The neighbors contacted my mom and asked me to babysit again. It happened again. I went home and did not tell my parents a thing. Finally, I refused to go back to my neighbor's house. Mom never knew why."

Janelle got married young and divorced quickly, but not before she had Jenny, the light of her life. The two shared a special bond.

When Jenny was about 6 years old, Janelle remarried. Her second husband, Dave, kept looking at Jenny inappropriately, walking in on her while she was in the bathroom or while she was dressing or undressing.

Soon into their marriage the couple had three children close together. While Janelle would take care of the three younger children, Dave would sit next to Jenny on the sofa watching television with a comforter over them and molest her.

Jenny says that, ironically, she, her mother and stepfather were becoming more active in the LDS church at the time.

Another Silent Victim

We are supposed to be doing my homework. I know mom will come in here and catch us. She's going to blame me. I'm the one. There must be something wrong with me that makes him do this. It's my fault that he touches me.

How can he do this here? I hope mom will come in. For God's sake we are right here in the living room. He's got my underwear down. His mouth is between my legs. I'm just going to close my eyes and hold my breath until he is finished. Hold my breath until I just stop breathing.

Dave started fondling and having oral sex with Jenny when she was 10 years old. He had been her stepfather for some years and just had another child with Jenny's mother, Janelle. The sexual abuse lasted almost three years.

"I knew what he was doing wasn't right. He made me feel that if I didn't go along with it, no one would love me," Jenny says. "I needed, more than anything else, to be loved."

Dave was bold in his perversion, feeling as if it was his right to take what he wanted when and where he wanted it.

"My girlfriend and I were showing him some photographs of us dancing," Jenny says. "We were both sitting on the living room floor and he just sat down between us and started molesting both of us. He put his hands in our shorts and we both sat there embarrassed and scared. We didn't say a thing."

The sexual abuse continued until her mother walked into the kitchen when Dave had his hands up Jenny's shirt. "I lost it," says Janelle. "I just flew at him."

Jenny says: "I was so ashamed, I ran up into my room and locked myself in. I didn't come out for the longest time."

Janelle started divorce proceedings and turned Dave into the police. He was convicted and spent just 3 months in jail. Jenny remembers the day he was released from jail. "He came right over to the house. He had this huge Cheshire cat grin. I wanted to smack it off his face. He knew he'd gotten away with it and now he was worming his way back into our family."

Janelle and Dave remarried. "I lost all respect for my mom," Jenny says. "I could not believe she was putting me back into that hell. I told her, *Just make sure you put a lock on my door!* I rebelled against her. I talked back to her. I was a terror as a teenager. I was promiscuous, I think just to get back at Dave."

The couple divorced again when Jenny was 16. "Mom just couldn't trust him and she didn't want to live that way anymore," Jenny says. Within a few years, Dave married an older single woman in the LDS temple.

When Jenny had her first child, Dave visited her and Janelle, bringing with him and gloating over his Mormon wife and their 2-year-old son. Jenny sat silent watching in horror as Janelle allowed Dave to hold her newborn. Dave's power over Janelle and Jenny was palatable. The sickness cast an eerie shadow in the room as he beamed with patriarchal pride, claiming his place as grandfather over Jenny's son.

"He doesn't deserve to be part of my life," Jenny says. "He is not going to be in my children's lives!" The next time Dave tried to give her son a birthday present, Jenny went to his proper LDS home and threw the gift in his face.

No Child Is Safe

Janelle found, unfortunately, that her second daughter wasn't safe from molesters either. Kari was in 6th grade when "Officer Friendly" began to stalk her. The Layton policeman visited elementary schools, teaching and preaching about dangerous strangers. Officer Friendly paid too much attention to Kari and people were starting to notice. He would target Kari as the child that he would put on his lap, out of all the children in the class. He started showing back up to Kari's elementary school, when school let out for the day.

Mom, being a victim herself, noticed more and more how much Officer Friendly was in her child's personal space. At first Janelle thought that maybe she was being too protective.

70

After some detective work on her part, Janelle became convinced that this police officer was molesting her daughter. She was furious. "Hell no! Over my dead body!" She cried and held Kari. Then she dried her tears and got busy. She got her reports, documents and concrete evidence together and declared a war on another one of Utah's child molesters. She reported Officer Friendly to his superiors at the Layton Police Department. They did nothing.

Officer Friendly continued molesting little girls over and over again for about seven more years until there were just too many complaints and reports for police to ignore. He was finally convicted. But what about all of those little girls?

Janelle doesn't pull any punches when it comes to the LDS church: "Sexual abuse is all too common here. It has to do with our religion, with this culture and mentality. Bishops who are aware, who have been told that this is going on with a family member in the ward, in my opinion, they are legally responsible to report it. So many priesthood leaders think. *well, we don't want this to get out, so let's handle it ourselves.* It gets swept under the rug and another child is sacrificed in the name of Mormonism."

Janelle continues: "These priesthood holders think they have all this mighty power that they can change a pedophile, that everything will be all right just as long as he repents. They close their eyes to what they don't want to see and close their ears to what they don't want to hear."

(Author's Note: Any human being. I don't care what religion you are, I don't give a damn what position you hold in the community or any church, as a human being, a human person, you have the responsibility to stand up for these children and punish the perpetrators.)

The Body Rebels

Janelle has been diagnosed with fibromyalgia and is on several medications including Paxil for depression and anxiety. Is it merely coincidental that most women with fibromyalgia are victims of childhood molestation and rape?

Fibromyalgia is a cluster of symptoms including deep muscle pain, piercing headaches, severe fatigue and mental confusion sometimes referred to as "fibro-fog." Physicians treat the syndrome with Elavil, to encourage restorative sleep.

The treatment is a panacea, at best. There is no cure. Many people with fibromyalgia can only work at something for about two hours then they are exhausted and must rest. The body aches everyday from head to toe.

Kathy Lewis, a Canadian survivor of ritual abuse and child prostitution who suffers from fibromyalgia, says one of the most devastating effects of childhood sexual abuse comes from being told over and over again that what is happening isn't really happening, that what hurts doesn't hurt. This destroys the victim's ability to trust their own senses, to take care of themselves and listen to their bodies. Children taught to ignore both physical and emotional pain, suffer exceedingly as adults when that pain rebels and asserts its right to be felt.

Lewis says that survivors must monitor the amount of time they can function and when they need rest. They must protect themselves and become selfish with their time, and their emotional and physical output. Survivors need a circle of friends and family whom they can turn to when a life of pain becomes too much. Friends and family members must understand that sometimes survivors are not going to meet their obligations. They will have a few good days and many very bad days.

The headaches, muscle pain and fatigue of fibromyalgia are constant and life altering, Lewis says. Living with left over pain from abuse can limit the life of adults molested as children. It can leave them susceptible to alcoholism, drug abuse or suicide to kill the pain that they cannot convince others is real. People, even the most understanding, may think survivors are making it up or seeking attention. This is extremely damaging to the person with fibromyalgia. Any pain survivors feel must be acknowledged and respected by the victim and by the people she trusts and loves.

Grandma's Favorite

Ever since I can remember, grandma has been doing this. Putting me in the bathtub, washing me all over, even after I started growing hair between my legs. Now, I'm drunk, throwing up in the toilet and I really need her. She's taking my clothes off to get into the bathtub. The water is warm and I'm feeling a little better.

Like always, grandma is washing me everywhere. Now, she's drying me off. Now, she's sucking my penis.

Kirk remembers that his grandma was "a cuddly kind of person" and would come into the bathroom to see if he washing properly. "I felt sort of odd being 12 years old and having to be washed up by my grandma. I didn't tell her to stop or anything even if I felt weird about it," Kirk says. After the night she forced oral sex on Kirk, "she's been fucking me all the time. We never talk about having sex, we just do it."

I talked with Kirk when he was 14 and in residential day treatment for behavior problems and severe depression.

"It seemed so common for me to be naked with my grandma," Kirk says. "She would tickle me all over with her tongue. I love her, I mean I'm in love with her. My grandma used to tell me all the time that we were going to get married some day. We would stay at home a lot and she would have sex with me." Before Kirk began day treatment for depression, he didn't have many friends. He lived with his grandmother, who has legal custody of him.

Would your grandmother ask you to have sex with her? How would you and she get to that point?

"No, she would just be around me, near me, when nobody else was around."

What would she do?

"Just sit around me!"

Would she say anything?

"Sometimes, you know she would just grab my cock and say come here. Then she would start blowing me off. Then I would fuck her."

When was the last time you saw your grandma?

"I had a weekend visit a couple of days ago."

Would you mind telling me about your visit?

"Yeah, I can tell you about it. She picked me up Friday, signed me out after talking to the social worker, gave me a hug saying that I'm getting so big. We left. While in the car, she asked if I missed her. I said yes and that's when she put her hand on my thigh. She said, I sure did miss you! Then she slid her hand up to the elastic of my sweat pants."

73

What did she do then?

>*"She put her right hand on my penis and started rubbing on it and was getting me hard like jacking me off. She said I can't wait to get you home mmmmmm."*

Did the two of you go straight home?

>*"No. She pulled into the 7-Eleven and she asked me if I wanted anything. She gave me a $10 bill so I went in and got some soda and some candy and stuff. Oh, I forgot, some girls in the car we pulled up next to saw that I had a boner and laughed and pointed at it."*

Were you embarrassed?

>*"Yeah."*

Did you and your grandma go home then?

>*"Yeah."*

Do you want to continue talking or do you want a break?

>*"We can keep talking if you want."*

So you two got home?

>*"Oh, yeah, I was kind of nervous 'cause in therapy we talked about incest. You know, having sex with a relative and stuff like that."*

Then what happened when you got inside the house?

>*"I went to the living room took my shoes off and was watching television then grandma came back in."*

Where did she go?

>*"I think she went to her room 'cause she came back with her robe on with her house shoes on. She sat down next to me while I was watching TV and put her hand on my neck."*

What do you mean, what part of your neck?

>*"She had her hand on like the back of my neck playing with my hair. She wanted to know what I wanted for dinner."*

What did she do then?

>*"She watched TV with me then she went to cook. I could tell that she didn't have anything on under her robe because she didn't have the snaps together on the bottom part."*

Did the two of you talk about anything while you were sitting on the couch?

>*"Yeah, yeah. She asked me about what I talked about in therapy and I told her that they don't like us to talk about what we talk about in therapy sessions."*

74

What did your grandma say to that?

"She rubbed my chest and put her hand on my penis and was smiling and said, Oh you can talk to grandma about anything. You don't have to worry about grandma saying anything to anybody, OK?"

So did you tell her about your therapy conversations?

"Yeah, then I asked her about it."

About what?

"About having sex with people in my family."

What did you ask her exactly, do you remember?

"Yeah, I asked her if what we were doing was wrong because in therapy they said it was not right, that it was incest."

What did she say then?

"She asked me if I told the therapist about what we do."

And?

"I told her that I was supposed to be open and honest so I talked about it."

What did she say?

"She asked me if I loved her. I said, Yeah."

What did she say then?

"She said that's all that matters because she loves me, too. Then she told me to go take a shower and get ready for dinner."

Do you know how old your grandmother is?

"I think she's about 60."

So what did she fix for dinner?

"Oh, she made my favorite, pork chops, mashed potatoes and corn on the cob. It was good, too."

So what did you do after dinner?

"I played on my play station until she said it was time to go to bed. I looked in my room. There were no sheets or anything on my bed."

What happened then?

"She came up behind me and told me that my sheets and stuff were dirty and I could sleep with her in her bed. So I went into her room with her. Grandma told me that she wanted me to give her a hug and kiss goodnight."

Were you still dressed in your clothes?

"No, I had on my robe and underwear."

Where was your grandma?

"She was over by her dresser so I went over to her and we were kissing. She pulled off my robe and took my underwear off while she was kissing and licking me all over my body. She let her robe drop off. We were butt naked."

Was she making all the sexual advances?

"No."

Did you kiss and feel her body, too?

"Yeah, it always felt good. I liked it."

Then what happened?

"She was giving me head and I was rubbing her hair and boobs. Then we were on the bed and she was teaching me how to give her oral sex."

Did you learn what she wanted you to learn?

"Yeah. She told me that I was doing a good job."

Did you have intercourse with her, too?

"Oh yeah. We always do that. We did it in the shower on Saturday, too. Then we went to the mall to get me some new tennis shoes."

Are those your new shoes?

"Yeah," he said, smiling.

How long have you been in therapy?

"About six months."

Do you have any problems about having sex with your grandma?

"Yeah, I'm worried because I think that I'm going to have to go to a foster home and they won't let me go back to live with my grandma."

What are your true feelings about incest?

"Well, in therapy they said it was wrong."

Do you think it's wrong?

"In a way because she's a relative. But I love my grandma and she loves me. What we're doing is wrong but we've been doing it since I was a kid."

Are you not stopping because she's your grandma and she loves you, or because it feels good and you're used to it?

"It's all that I am used to. It's like she's my girlfriend."

Is that normal and healthy to have your grandmother as your girlfriend?

"No."

76

Kirk sighed and looked away from me like he was embarrassed. Eye contact was quite limited after that.

At this point, Kirk is in foster care. Last I heard, his grandmother was still visiting him. It's important to note here that if the system doesn't take a stand and follow through when the therapist takes and submits notes, then the child is going to remain lost in a system of abuse and bureaucracy. Lost in the middle of rape and red tape, in the meantime growing older day by day, with all these bad habits, all these aberrant behaviors, conditioning the child into a certain kind of adult and parent. When a victim goes through this year after year, society has another concern. With all that baggage, the victim has got to empty it out on something or somebody.

When he grows up, the victim will have to work through his feelings in therapy or, statistics show, he will turn his frustrations on to other children and do what was done to him.

Boys Are Victims, Too

Judging from the many male perpetrators in the LDS church and in Utah, it is most likely that these adult male predators are former child victims themselves.

The dynamic of male sexual abuse demands secrecy. Boys are socialized at an early age to believe any sexual experience, at any age, with a girl or woman is man-making and a rite of passage. And when abused by a male, the shame of perceived homosexuality is so great that boys rarely tell.

Forced, coerced and premature sex by any female with power over a boy can cause confusion, depression and rage. Boys are socialized to be "macho," demanding that they not let themselves be victims or even vulnerable. Boys are children. They are weaker than their perpetrators. Child molesters are usually stronger physically and more knowledgeable. They know how to manipulate and control a child.

Many male victims feel deep guilt and shame when they experience arousal while being abused. Child abusers use a boy's natural sexual response against him. The predator can maintain secrecy by telling the child that his response means he is a willing participant and likes the activity.

Physical response, erection and ejaculation, often happens even in painful and traumatic sexual situations. It does not mean the boy desires the experience or even understands what it means. Boys abused by males may believe that something about them sexually attracts men, and that this might mean they are effeminate or homosexual. The pedophile's inability to develop a healthy adult sexual relationship is the problem – not the physical features of an immature boy. Most child molesters who seek out boys are not homosexual. They are pedophiles.

A majority of pedophiles do have histories of being sexually abused themselves. There is a primary difference between sexual abuse victims who perpetrate and those who never perpetrate. Those who do not go on to hurt other children told someone about the abuse. These victims were believed and supported by significant people in their lives. They were given the help they needed to heal. That makes all the difference.

No Safe Haven

I just got out of the bath. He's putting the shiny lotion all over me, spending a lot of time down there, where he puts his fingers inside me. I cry out in pain and he gives me warm milk to make me go to sleep. Then, I'm groggy, he gets on top of me and sticks it in. This isn't right, my uncle having sex with me. He treats me like his wife. My great-aunt doesn't know. If she knew she would stop him. Wouldn't she?

Sheri is now 46 years old. She was raped from the age of 6 to 16. The pedophile primed this toddler with his fingers and shortly thereafter forced sexual intercourse. She escaped the torture when she was 16, marrying an older man so she didn't have to go back to the house of pain. Unfortunately, she married an abuser. Her husband raped her 15-year-old daughter. Sheri's daughter had two children by this man.

Diagnosed with Lupus, Sheri has serious physical and mental illnesses. She's had gynecological problems since she was 8 as a direct result of rape at an early age. She has been hospitalized six times for psychological evaluation.

Difficulties with relationships abound with her three daughters and one son, who has been in prison since he was a teen. Dealing with the opposite sex poses serious problems since her history with men has been hellish. Sheri lives alone and is often so sick physically that she is only out of bed to eat and go to the bathroom. This sometimes lasts for days.

Tell me about your earliest memory of your foster father?

"I never lived with my biological parents. I lived with my great-aunt and her husband. My great-aunt must not have been at home when he was putting me to bed. I remember him putting the shiny lotion all over my body. He would spend a lot of time on and around my genitals. I would cry when he put his fingers inside of me. He would give me warm milk at bedtime. The warm milk always helped me to calm down."

Why do you think you remember the warm milk?

"I found out, as time went by, that he had been giving me sleeping pills to keep me under control while he raped me."

How old were you the first time he fully raped you?

"I was close to 7 years old. He would tell me not to tell and bribe me with gifts. He told me he loved me, not my great-aunt. It was like I was his woman, his wife."

Did you tell anyone about the abuse?

"One day while I was in class, the school counselor called me into her office to meet with a social worker. She knew something was wrong. I still didn't admit it."

Did anyone do anything to help you?

"My grandma and aunt confronted him. They were arguing loudly and I recall him saying that he was going to leave. Then my aunt saying he didn't have to go. He stopped raping me for about a year. Then he started up again. That's when I realized I had better get on birth control."

Did you tell your aunt that he started raping you again?

"No, I didn't want to have to go to a foster home and be separated from my brother. We were wards of the state. I was trying to get my own family and get married and move out. I think he would have continued to rape me for as long as I stayed in that house."

How has being raped for 10 years affected your life?

"I've had numerous female problems for most of my life. I've been admitted to the hospital six times for psychiatric problems. My life is basically a mess."

Sheri does believe there is hope for victims. "Tell someone about the abuse. Tell and tell again until someone listens and stops the abuser," she says.

Family Affairs

Oh, just shut up. You know you like it. Open your legs. Just one last time for good luck. C'mon, you know you're going to miss it. I'm leaving tomorrow on my mission. Let me fuck you while I can. You're going to miss me, sis.

Annette remembers being molested by her parents and raped by her two brothers from 4 years old until she left home at 18. The wealthy family was active in the LDS church. Her father is a stake president, a leader over several congregations, called "wards." Her brother raped her before he left on his mission.

Annette's parents molested her in the family jacuzzi. Her two brothers, both two years older than her and each other, were often included in the naked bath molestation sessions. When the parents finished sodomizing them and making them do unspeakable things to each other, they sent the kids to bed.

"After a few minutes the boys would come into my bedroom," Annette says. "They would take me out of my little princess bed and rape me until they got tired or bored. I just thought this was normal behavior. I didn't know anything else."

She particularly dreaded Sunday because there was more free time for her parents and brothers to assault her.

"Mom would get us up in the morning, if we weren't already in bed with them, and tell us she was going to help us get dressed for church," Annette says. "Mom and dad were married in the temple. That was special because it meant they could become gods after they died and we would be with them for eternity. An eternal family."

An Elitist Attitude

The family saw themselves as being above or better than other people. "People of color were never allowed inside our home because they are cursed," Annette says. "I met a black girl who was one of a handful who attended our high school. She was very nice and smart. A lot of the kids in my school were prejudice against Indian, blacks, Spanish-speaking and Asian kids. They would tease and torment them every day especially on the way to seminary." Seminary is a Mormon "bible class" junior high and high school students take during school hours.

Annette recalls an incident that remains seared into her mind. "One day the football team came into the girls' locker room and cornered an Asian girl who was showering after gymnastic practice. I hid in a corner across the room. I just froze. I held my own mouth shut to stop myself from screaming.

"There were like eight to ten boys. They raped her. They wouldn't stop. They did it for about an hour. I just couldn't move. They would scream *Yahoo!* every time they ejaculated in her, or on her, or near her. It was just unbelievable. I couldn't believe this was happening. Some of them were jacking off as they waited for their turn. Ever since then, I hate it whenever I hear somebody say *Yahoo!* My brothers told me to stay away from *niggers, spiks and chinks*. They never gave me a good reason why. I never heard anything about the locker room gang rape. I was too afraid to say anything to anyone until now. What a load off my mind."

After the gang rape, Annette said she cried all the way home, went to bed without dinner and was awakened at about 10 p.m. by her bother who wanted to rape her one last time for "good luck" before he left for his mission.

This mission business is expected of young men right after they graduate high school. They go out into the world and spread Mormon doctrine. With them goes everything they learned at home. "We all got up the next morning, ate a big breakfast then piled into the family van and took him to the airport," she says. "I will miss my big brother. There is a part of me that loves him. I was so sad that night, mom and dad had sex with me and rocked me to sleep. The next day, my parents went to the temple to pray for his safe return."

Annette says the special underwear or "garments" that her parents and, now her brothers, wear have a repulsive meaning for her. "There were slits or openings in the right places, you know what I mean. My parents never took their garments off when they raped me. Garments open at the crotch, it was easy access for them," she says. "My parents always told us that *what happens in this house, stays in this house.*"

Annette is about to attend college: "I want to study social work and help people. I think I can be good at it."

Polygamy's Daughter

At first I thought this was a funny game. My brothers tied me to the bunk bed like they were robbers. Now, they are hurting me. They're taking my clothes off. They are putting their hands and mouths and private parts on me. I can't cry hard enough. I don't like this. They say it's my fault. They say to keep my mouth shut or they will tell mom that I started it. They say she will beat me. I know she will. I promise I won't tell.

Linda, a 34-year-old white single mother of four, was raped by her three older brothers from the time she was 6 to 8 years old. She is the 7th of 11 children, a daughter of a polygamist who had five wives and a total of 36 children.

"My brothers forced sexual intercourse, they raped me, made me jack them off and made me let them lick me," Linda says. "It was a nightmare. They said I deserved it. They said my mom would beat me if I told her. They were right."

Linda told her aunts, her mother and her father about the rapes when she was 7 years old. "Sure enough, my mom beat me and told me it was my fault. Nobody did anything to help me. No matter how many times I told someone, they said I was lying. They told me I would go to hell. They said I had an active imagination or a bad dream. They said it didn't happen."

A few years ago, at a family reunion, Linda attacked one of her brothers after he covertly assaulted her. "He came up to me, gave me a hug, put his hand down my shirt and grabbed my nipple. I shoved his head right into a tree, lodged it in there between two limbs. They had to cut up the tree to get him out.

82

"I still have so much anger from what happened to me as a child. Sometimes I don't know what to do with it," she says.

What she doesn't do is take it out on her own children. Linda has cultivated an open and loving relationship with her four kids chiefly because her own parents did not protect her. She currently has custody of a son and daughter.

"Now that I have children of my own, I listen to what they tell me very carefully and let them know that they can discuss anything with me," Linda says. "So far we have a great relationship. We have discussed many topics including my childhood. I let them know if anyone tries to hurt them or do anything bad to them even if they threaten them or me, they can tell me about it and I will believe them."

Linda says: "Sexual abuse is all too common in the state of Utah. It's a terrible thing when it happens and no one breaks the cycle. The Mormon church stifles the kids and their sexual development. They can't have sex or experiment with their peers in any healthy way so they turn to family members in secret."

Ritualized Abuse

A 3M enters the room with three of his seven daughters as they walk reverently toward what appears to be an alter made ready for the cleansing ritual. My feet are bare. The floor should be cold. I can't feel it. I don't care. Look ahead at the hem of the white robe in front. Walk. I am one of the chosen few. Smile. We stand close together, very close. Clothing is removed. The anointing with oil. Prayers and chants. The washings begin.

Say nothing. Soon it will be over I know what happens to those who protest. They . . . disappear. What is happening? I should feel pain. The knife. The shocks. The probing. I can't feel it. I don't care. I am beyond numb. No matter. The children inside my head are dancing now, taking me away, twisting, twirling, flying free. Away from here.

"Basically, everyone just thinks we're crazy," Crystal says. "And maybe they are right. If I am crazy, it's not my fault. It's theirs, the abusers."

Crystal grew up in an LDS family, married in the temple and lived the life of a typical stay-at-home Mormon wife with a husband and five children. They all attended church together. She went visiting teaching, sharing religious messages with other women of the church and helping them with home life. After the birth of her last daughter, Crystal packed a bag and left.

"I couldn't ignore the images in my head," she says. "Something evil, unspeakable happened to me as a child. I had to get away. I couldn't stay." She saw the images play over and over again: A group of men in white robes touching her, washing her body, anointing her with oil, raping her, using electric shock torture on her genitals, chanting words and phrases as they showed her in graphic detail how she would die if she told.

"This kind of abuse involves sexual molestation and rape. They use mind control, physical, spiritual, mental and emotional manipulation. They do this deliberately to create a split in the person so that the split is forced into perpetrating," Crystal says. "Some people are more difficult to split than others. They are worked on extra."

Crystal says the "light-of-day" person has no idea that he or she has a split that is a perpetrator. "The occurrences sound so far fetched that when we start to remember, we don't tell anyone. This is changing. We are at a point in history, and evolution, where hidden things are being brought to light."

Inside families like Crystal's, ritual abuse is often generational and deeply hidden from neighbors and co-workers. Survivor accounts also relate the existence of secret societies inside secret societies, where factions of fraternal organizations, church congregations, and government agencies are actively involved in overt destructive occult activities. Many victims report they had their first flashbacks of ritual abuse when they went through the LDS temple the first time.

When Crystal started experiencing personality disorders associated with ritualistic abuse, she sought support from *Mr. Light & Associates, Inc.* located in Ogden, Utah. The non-profit organization offers ritual abuse education and victim services.

In some localities the ritualistic abuse groups appear to adopt the beliefs of the most dominant religion – such as the Mormons in Utah, says Jeanne Adams, founder of *Mr. Light & Associates, Inc.*

84

At the same time, ritualistic pedophiles infiltrate positions of respect within those religious communities, Adams says. Ritual abuse victims often develop dissociate disorder in reaction to years of deep psychological and physical trauma. The disorder may be a simple blocking or forgetting. In severe situations of repeated, unacknowledged abuse, the formation of multiple personalities may result.

Within These Walls
In 1990, Mormon bishop Glenn L. Pace, a member of the LDS Strengthening Church Members Committee, said victims of ritualistic abuse reported to him that sometimes the abuse took place in Mormon churches.

"I have met with 60 victims. All 60 individuals are members of the church. The majority were abused by relatives, often their parents," Pace reported. "All have developed psychological problems and most were diagnosed with multiple personality disorder or some other dissociative disorder.

"Not only do some of the perpetrators represent a cross section of Mormon culture. Sometimes the abuse has taken place in our own meeting houses," Pace wrote.

About 25% of children molested or raped use dissociation for relief from chronic sexual abuse, says James Freisen, author of *Uncovering the Mystery of MPD*, published in 1991. "Some of these victims, develop Multiple Personal Disorder, now called Dissociative Identity Disorder. In comparison, ritual abuse is so much more terrible a kind of abuse that it causes dissociation in a much higher percentage of its victims, maybe as high as 75% or even more," Freisen wrote.

Dissociative Identity Disorder may include suicidal behavior, episodes of lost time or amnesia, abusive relationships in adulthood, strong attacks of shame, and being able to turn off pain or "put it out of the mind." Victims also may be involved in substance abuse and self-mutilation or self-injuring behavior. They may hear voices and have visual, auditory and somatic (body memory) flashbacks.

Other symptoms may include: phobia or panic attacks, substance abuse, seizure like episodes, sleep disorders, sleepwalking, psychic experiences, eating disorders, sexual difficulties and a history of multiple mental illness diagnoses.

They may be diagnosed with depression with suicide ideation, schizophrenia, bipolar disorder and/or borderline personality disorder. Many victims report odd changes or variations in physical skills and interests.

Crystal had another child by a different partner almost two years ago. She is raising her son alone as she sees fit, traveling in a van and making money as a licensed massage therapist. She has left the Mormon church and says God is helping her to heal her past and find peace.

"Victims need to know that what happened to us is not our fault. We do have a responsibility to stop the secret works," Crystal says. "We can heal. It's difficult, nearly impossible really, but it can be done."

Chapter 4

LDS Sacred or Sordid Secrets?

Talking with Mormons the past four years, I've found that there are many of them who don't know the details of their own religion. Many do not know the factual history, as opposed to folk tales, of the LDS church. They do not know the exact doctrine they profess to believe. If they do know, they rarely question these beliefs even if certain practices go against their intrinsic or intuitive understanding of right and wrong.

More than a religion, Mormonism is a tenaciously rooted way of life. This is how their families have lived for 170 years, following the beliefs and habits of their parents, grandparents, great-grandparents, for some as far back as 10 generations. Since they have babies relatively young, a Mormon generation is based on having a child every 20 years. Assuming Joseph Smith's descendents kept to this production schedule, Joe the 10th would be 12 years old this year.

On the outside, the LDS church looks almost too good to be true. Clean-cut children, modestly dressed, not smoking, not drinking, helpful as Scouts every one. Take a longer look and the façade begins to crumble.

Once a real conversation progresses, you can hear bones clinking as skeletons force their way out of barricaded closets.

What happens when these stringently molded children get on their own as young adults? Some do continue on the "straight and narrow" path they were told God wants them to follow. They achieve in school, they go on missions, they finish college, they marry in the temple as virgins, find financial success, bear three or more children and remain faithful to their spouse.

Reality check. When children are reared to blindly obey external rules set down by parents or by a religion, they have few opportunities to make choices for themselves. We all learn by making mistakes. Allowed to test our boundaries, slip up and learn from natural consequences *at a young age* is safer than waiting until the consequences increase in severity as we grow older.

For example, adolescents with freedom to make choices may learn that overindulgence in alcohol can make them sick and cause embarrassment. They don't go there again. If the first drink comes in his 20s fueled by rebellion and the Mormon hasn't learned for himself, he may get irresponsibly drunk and behind the wheel of a car. The consequence then won't be getting sick over the toilet but may well be killing himself or someone else.

Or an adolescent who has the freedom to experience natural sexual development responsibly without deep-seated guilt, may decide, "Hey, this feels good, but I don't want to be a parent, I don't want a sexually transmitted disease, I don't want to be entangled in this kind of intimacy at my age." Told to stay completely away from natural sexual inquiry because God will punish them or they will be locked out of the "celestial kingdom," when young Mormons are let loose to make choices for themselves, they often have no internal boundaries to help them make wise sexual decisions.

There's a phenomena that occurs with many LDS young people when they leave their sheltered homes and venture out on their own. *Many of them do not know who they are, what they stand for or what they believe apart from the church.* Often, they lack the basic experience or "hard knocks" to support their beliefs. They haven't learned life's lessons for themselves.

Freedom To Choose?

The Mormon church claims to give its members "free agency" to make their own choices. It seems however, they really only have the freedom to choose the church's position.

When a child is told, "Don't do this because God said so," the potential for exaggerated rebellion is set in place. Not only do young adult Mormons test the limits parents and the church set for them, they tend to go overboard. They have found a powerful tool to defy authority and step out on their own. Such late-found independence usually comes at a high price.

Take drug experimentation, for instance. Mormon kids are told to stay away from alcohol and illicit drugs at all costs. Of course, that's a wise idea. However, Mormon youths often don't have factual information to support that directive. Their drug (and sex) education is sorely lacking. And their behavior is based upon an external mandate, instead of an internal understanding. They haven't yet made a personal decision not to use drugs, they simply don't because they were told not to.

What if they decide to rebel or even just experiment: "I'm going to do the drug thing." Do they know they can become an alcoholic through excessive, irresponsible drinking? Do they know inhalants can kill them on the first try and cause brain damage if used repeatedly? That regular marijuana use can become a monkey on their backs if they use it to numb uncomfortable feelings, escape guilt or avoid the normal responsibilities of life? Do they know acid (or LSD) can hardwire them for psychological breaks or mental illness? That they will irreversibly kill brain cells if they drop Ecstacy? Or is their behavior fueled only by a need to disrespect their parents and rebel against an oppressive church? Do they know they can become physically addicted to methamphedamine or "speed," tranquilizers, heroine, crack or cocaine? Do they care? At that point, it may well be that their religious conditioning has damned them into believing that they deserve whatever punishment their actions bring.

The same thing happens with sex The majority of Mormons I've talked with, even those in adult relationships, do not use condoms to protect against pregnancy, or even more importantly against sexually transmitted diseases.

In their minds, incurable genital herpes, fertility threatening chlamydia, and even AIDS only afflicts non-Mormons. Though most of them know very well what they're looking for, sexual relations, they claim to get "swept up" in the moment. Even after the first time, when they should learn from the mistake, these young people and mature adults continue to get swept up on a regular basis. They ignorantly maintain that they have no control over what happens in the sexual arena. They refuse to take responsibility for their sexual actions and decisions.

Pressured To Be Perfect

"Now, you know the rules, don't mess up!" Healthy people do not expect perfection from themselves or their children. The Mormon church is all about attaining, expecting and requiring perfection on Earth and in the afterlife.

In *Doctrines of Salvation*, (Vol.2, p.39), Joseph Fielding Smith Jr., wrote: "Sons of God become Gods. If the faithful, who keep the commandments of the Father, are his sons, then they are heirs of the kingdom and shall receive of the fullness of the Father's glory, even until they become like the Father. *And how can they be perfect as their Father in heaven is perfect if they are not like him.*"

The Mormon book of scripture, the *Doctrine & Covenants (chapter 128, verse 18)*, states: ". . . the earth will be smitten with a curse unless there is a welding link between fathers and children, (through) baptisms for the dead. *For we without them cannot be made perfect; neither can they without us be made perfect. Neither can they nor we be made perfect without those who have died in the gospel also;* for it is necessary *that a whole and complete and perfect union and welding together of dispensations,* should take place."

Perfectionism is a trap. The harder a person strives for perfection, the worse his or her disappointment, and in severe cases self-hate, will become. Perfection is an abstract concept that does not exist in the real world, and rightly so. People expecting perfection run into some huge problems in life which set them up for failure. They become afraid, nervous, unwilling to risk mistakes that are necessary for growth. They become highly self-critical. They don't allow themselves to enjoy their successes because no matter how well they do, it is not good enough. It is never perfect because it never can be.

90

Perfectionism makes people intolerant of others. They may not have many real friends, they may feel resentment from family members and children, because people don't appreciate being judged and nagged.

The perfectionist is so afraid of making mistakes that he or she doesn't venture to try new things or take risks that might lead to new discoveries. Perfectionism narrows their world, makes them bored and restless, constantly asking themselves, isn't there something more to life?

Obey Without Question

On Nov. 9, 1997, an Australian journalist interviewed current LDS president Gordon B. Hinckley, asking him if church members have the freedom to question doctrine and practices. A portion of the interview follows: Does there not seem to be an uncritical acceptance of a conformist style in your church?

Hinckley: Uncritical? No. Not uncritical. People think in a very critical way before they come into this church. When they come into this church they're expected to conform. And they find happiness in that conformity.

They're not allowed to question?

Hinckley: Oh, they are allowed to question. Look, this church came of intellectual dissent. We maintain the largest private university in America, (Brigham Young University located in Provo, Utah) with 27,000 students.

And that dissent continues to this day?

Hinckley: Oh absolutely, absolutely. We expect people to think for themselves. Now, if they get off and begin to fight the church and that sort of thing as one or two do now and again, we simply disfellowship them and go our way. But those cases are really very, very few.

Oh, Mr. Hinckley, not true. Excommunication is used like an ax to cut down anyone who looks too closely at the church. For example, on Oct. 2, 1993, the *Salt Lake Tribune* reported the mass excommunication of six Mormon historians, authors and scholars. They are now known as the "September Six."

The *Tribune* article reads in part: "Three men and three women have been charged with apostasy for their writing and speaking about Mormon church subjects. The results?

91

"Paul Toscano, Avraham Gileadi, D. Michael Quinn, Maxine Hanks and Lavina Anderson were excommunicated. Lynne Whitesides was disfellowshiped. During the bishop's court or council, Whitesides was accused of *creating friction* with her Mormon feminist statements on television. Anderson was excommunicated for a single article in the independent Mormon journal, *Dialogue.* Her article, *The LDS Intellectual Community and Church Leadership* chronicled episodes of intimidation against Mormon historians and intellectuals for 20 years.

"Quinn, a respected LDS historian, has had three such councils within the last four months. He didn't attend the court: *I vowed I would never again participate in a process which was designed to punish me for being the messenger of unwanted historical evidence and to intimidate me from further work in Mormon history, Quinn said.*

"Gileadi, a conservative theologian, was excommunicated for his writings about the Apocalypse and Book of Isaiah. Some of those who were excommunicated used to write articles for the church's official publication, *The Ensign.* Quinn has written at least six articles for the magazine, and the same number for *Brigham Young University Studies.* "

In *Faithful History,* a book written by Quinn, the author recalls an intellectual run-in with Mormon apostle Boyd K. Packer: "When Elder Packer interviewed me as a prospective member of Brigham Young University's faculty in 1976, he explained: *I have a hard time with historians because they idolize the truth. The truth is not uplifting; it destroys. I could tell most of the secretaries in the church office building they are ugly and fat. That would be the truth, but it would hurt and destroy them. Historians should tell only that part of the truth that is inspiring and uplifting.* "

In a 1981 speech, Packer made these comments: "There is a temptation for the writer or the teacher of church history to want to tell everything, whether it is worthy or faith promoting or not. Some things that are true are not very useful."

On May 26, 1945, the Ward Teachers Message, printed in the *Deseret News*, Church Section p. 5, discouraged members from questioning their beliefs:

"When our leaders speak, the thinking has been done. When they propose a plan, it is God's Plan. When they point the way, there is no other which is safe. When they give directions, it should mark the end of controversy. God works in no other way. To think otherwise, without immediate repentance, may cost one his faith, destroy his testimony, and leave him a stranger to the kingdom of God."

92

Every church should welcome scrutiny. All religions are manmade. If the principles are solid, the church should be open to members and non-members asking questions about doctrine, policies, practices and history. In fact, such research is necessary to cement a personal religious understanding and belief.

The late LDS president, Marion G. Romney, said in a Conference Report October 1960: "Always keep your eye on the president of the church, and if he ever tells you to do anything, *even if it is wrong, and you do it*, the Lord will bless you for it but you don't need to worry. The Lord will never let his mouthpiece lead you astray."

Even if it is wrong, you won't be held responsible? Does this sound familiar? History has proven over and over again what happens when people follow blindly without questioning authority. Unquestioned beliefs can destroy lives; Slavery. The Holocaust. Jim Jones and mass suicides in the name of God. The World Trade Towers massacre. In 1997, members of the religious cult Heaven's Gate killed themselves in San Diego, California, believing that after they died, a spaceship hiding behind the Hale-Bopp comet nearing Earth would take them to heaven.

In the 21st Century, when we should be an enlightened and educated people, millions of Mormons still accept doubtful practices, strange rituals and peculiar requests with blinders on. Most people outside of Utah don't think or act that way anymore. I'm convinced that the Mormon Mecca is at least 40 to 50 years behind the rest of the nation.

Are Mormons Christians?

The LDS church recently demanded that the media drop the "Mormon" designation and use only *The Church of Jesus Christ of Latter-day Saints*, in an attempt to come across as a mainstream Christian church, especially during worldwide coverage of the 2002 Winter Olympic Games in February.

Mormons practice a religion very different from traditional Christianity. In particular, they teach that God was once "as man is now." The LDS God progressed in knowledge and power to become a divine being with a perfect, resurrected body of flesh and bone. God has a wife, whom Mormons quietly refer to as their Heavenly Mother. Strangely enough members have been excommunicated or warned not to speak of her and definitely not to pray to her or even mention her in prayers.

93

The Mormon understanding of Jesus Christ is different from other Christian faiths. In Mormon doctrine, as God's firstborn spirit son, Jesus is the Jehovah of the Old Testament as well as the New Testament savior. Christ is also the only man physically begotten by God and his human mother, Mary, according the LDS doctrine. Stephen Robinson, a professor of religion at Brigham Young University was quoted as saying: *"Jesus has 46 chromosomes like everyone else. Twenty-three of those are from his Heavenly Father and 23 are from Mary."*

Christian fundamentalist religions oppose Mormonism as a cult. The Vatican recently ruled that Catholic converts from the LDS church must be re-baptized. It seems, the Pope does not consider Mormons to be Christian. Protestants, Presbyterians and Methodists also reject LDS baptisms as bogus. Mormons are baptized at the age of 8 or the age of their conversion by immersion into water by an LDS priesthood holder.

Mormons, of course, claim all other churches are untrue.

If a child is told in one breath that they belong to a Christian church and is led by priesthood members who claim God's inspiration, then they are abused by those men – the child becomes deeply psychologically, emotionally and spiritually confused. *So, does God want this to happen to me?* How is a 5-year-old supposed to rationalize or understand that?

While working in a residential day treatment facility for children in Salt Lake City, I noticed little kids 6, 7 and 8 years old, children who should be outside playing with their friends and having fun. During my tour of the facility, I asked, "Why are those little ones here? Oh, don't tell me, they aren't patients are they?" The answer was an unbelievable, "Yes!" The place was at capacity, they couldn't take anymore children. I had to ask the question: What's happening in this society that their very young children are so depressed and out of control that they need structured, professional therapy?

If there is no adequate intervention, many of these tiny victims will grow up to be victimized again and again, or enter adulthood with destructive behavior patterns and some will become adults who take on the role of perpetrator. At the least, their normal childhood development is disrupted, and now little children have to piece together their lives.

Modern Revelation

The same Australian journalist who interviewed Hinckley about conformity in the church also asked him about modern revelation. Mormons believe their modern-day "prophet" speaks directly to God and/or Jesus Christ, face-to-face if he wishes. Hinckley's answer is curious. Maybe, the leader didn't want to readily admit he talks intimately with the Almighty. After all, many people who claim they see God and talk with him one-on-one get committed to mental hospitals. I've interviewed some of these patients first hand. A portion of the journalist's interview follows: As the world leader of the church, how are you in touch with God? Can you describe that for me?

Hinckley: I pray. I pray to him. Night and morning, I speak with him. I think he hears my prayers. As he hears the prayers of others, I think he answers them.

But more than that, because you're a leader of the church, do you have a special connection?

Hinckley: I have a special relationship in terms of the church as an institution. Yes.

And you receive . . .?

Hinckley: For the entire church.

And you receive?

Hinckley: Now we don't need a lot of continuing revelation. We have a great, basic reservoir of revelation. But if a problem arises, as it does occasionally, a vexatious thing with which we have to deal, we go to the Lord in prayer. We discuss it as a First Presidency and as a Council of the Twelve Apostles. We pray about it and then come the whisperings of a still small voice. And we know the direction we should take and we proceed accordingly.

And this is a Revelation?

Hinckley: This is a Revelation.

How often have you received such revelations?

Hinckley: Oh, I don't know. I feel satisfied that in some circumstances we've had such revelation. It's a very sacred thing that we don't like to talk about it a lot.

But it's a special experience?

Hinckley: I think it's a real thing. It's a very real thing and a special thing. And a special experience.'

The *Book of Mormon*

Historians point out that the *Book of Mormon* describes a civilization lasting a thousand years in North and South America. The people of this region supposedly used horses, elephants, cattle, sheep, wheat, barley, steel, wheeled vehicles, shipbuilding, sails, coins, and other elements of Old World culture. But *not one artifact* of any of these common things has been found in the Americas of that period, historians say.

Nor does the *Book of Mormon* mention any features of the civilizations that did exist at that time in the Americas. The majority of key religions can substantiate Old World claims, geographically, archeologically and historically. Why not Mormonism? In fact, the history and civilization described in the *Book of Mormon* doesn't correspond to anything found by archaeologists anywhere in the Americas. I think this would concern a few Mormons, whose religion is based chiefly upon the *Book of Mormon*.

Historians tell us that the *Book of Mormon* claims to detail the religious and secular history of the inhabitants of the Western Hemisphere from about 2200 B.C. to about 421 A.D. These scriptures tell the reader that the American Indians or "Lamanites" are descended from immigrants who were led by God from their homes in the Near East to America. One group supposedly came from the Tower of Babel, and two other groups from *Jerusalem* just before the Babylonian Captivity, about 600 B.C. Historians argue whereas the *Book of Mormon* tells of a homogeneous people, with a single language, the pre-Columbian *history* of the Americas shows the opposite: Widely disparate racial types almost entirely east Asian (definitely not Semitic) who speak many unrelated languages, none connected to Hebrew or Egyptian.

Women In The Church

Maxine Hanks, excommunicated Mormon and editor of *Women and Authority: Re-emerging Mormon Feminism*, has said: "The extreme gender imbalance in Mormonism re-emerges in Utah's sexist culture, where government, education and business are run by Mormon men . . . In Utah, women as well as men repress the feminine, starve it and then overcompensate: *We crave sweet and fatty foods for comfort; we gain weight to feel loved; men act effeminate and women self-destruct with prescription drugs, obesity, depression and too many kids.*"

96

Hanks told the *Los Angeles Times* in an article published July 10, 1994: "The historical relationship of men and women in the Mormon church is a conflicted one . . . Mormon women exercised considerable religious authority in the LDS Church for 100 years and maintained some autonomy for 140 years.

"From 1830 to 1850, women received authority for blessings, healing and prophecy; priesthood keys, powers and rituals; and missionary calls. Women clashed with male leadership and lost authority at the turn of the century and again in the 1970s. Since 1991, Mormon feminists have encountered a backlash against attempts to reclaim women's authority. Today's church holds that women cannot exercise the priesthood, therefore women are not *ordained* only *set-apart* to church positions. As a full-time LDS missionary, I sensed I had the priesthood, but spent 19 months being denied the right to use t."

The church claims women cannot hold the priesthood because their "earthly calling" is to be mothers and raise righteous children. In fact, the responsibility for rearing and teaching children rests mainly on the mother's shoulders. Being a wife and a mother is said to be an honor equal to the priesthood even though motherhood does not allow for Mormon women to make any official decisions in their church. Apparently, being a husband and father comes secondary to priesthood responsibilities tied to the church. Husbands active in church callings often are absent from the home. With church counsel to have the wife stay at home and have many children, the man is also extra busy making a living.

Mormon women, in theory, stand on a sacred pedestal. In reality, their early history of polygamy reduced women to mere commodities. Historical documents quote LDS president Heber C. Kimball's opinion of women: *"I think no more of taking another wife than I do of buying a cow."*

During a recent interview with Hinckley, *"60 Minutes"* reporter Mike Wallace asked specifically about the priesthood, male-domination and complaints about child sexual abuse. A portion of the interview follows:

"Wallace: Fact is most Mormon women don't want to be priests. They accept that men control the church and dominate Mormon society. *And this has triggered complaints about how the church handles child sexual abuse.* A study has found that Mormon women who went to their clergyman for help believe the clergy were just not sympathetic.

"A sociologist tells us, at the root of the problem is that Mormon men have authority over women, so clergymen tend to sympathize with the men, the abusers, instead of the abused.

"Hinckley: That's one person's opinion. I, I don't think there's any substance to it. Now, there'll be a blip here, a blip there, a mistake here, a mistake there. But by and large, the welfare of women and children is as seriously considered as is the welfare of the men, if not more so."

Despite Hinckley's insistence that the church does not favor perpetrators, the history of Utah law and Mormon opinion shows differently. In 1992, senator Delpha Baird, a Republican from Holladay, expressed her anger at being excluded from a new state task force on treating Utah's sex offenders. The *Salt Lake Tribune* published a story on the controversy: "'I have great concern they need to have women's views on this because the majority of victims are female,' Baird said. In fact, there was only one woman appointed to the eight-person task force. Task force member and volunteer prison counselor, Duayne T. Johnson, said women don't show sex offenders enough compassion: *'One thing you'll find about women is they are so unforgiving for something like this that it becomes unreasonable.'*

"Senator Haven Barlow, a Layton Republican and head of the task force, agreed with Johnson. Barlow criticized mandatory minimum sentences for sex offenders. 'We have a mentality on sex offenders in this state that reminds me of some of the witch-hunt hysteria,' said Barlow, a Mormon who served as a volunteer religious counselor at the Utah State Prison at that time."

Demanding that child molesters and rapists be punished for their crimes is not "hysteria." Pedophilia is nearly impossible to treat successfully. Incarceration and mandatory mental health treatment are usually the only ways to keep these predators from hurting our children.

Mormon "Celestial" Marriage

LDS doctrine of eternal marriage in the temple makes it difficult, if not impossible, for a Mormon wife to obtain a divorce in the church, called a "temple divorce." A woman who attended church near my home, divorced her husband because he had become addicted to child pornography on the internet. This woman was frightened for her two young daughters.

Both she and her husband were returned missionaries. Since she filed for the divorce, her temple recommend was revoked. Without *proof* of sin, he could still attend the temple.

Mormon doctrine tells women that "divorce is usually the result of one or both not living the gospel," and that a woman who wants a divorce is "untrue to the covenants she has made in the house of the Lord." Legal civil divorces can be obtained fairly easily, but they create several problems in the religious life of a Mormon, writes Deborah Laake, the author of *Secret Ceremonies* who was excommunicated in 1993.

Laake writes, "After a civil divorce, a woman is considered unworthy to enter the temple, until she can prove to the heads of the church that the divorce was not caused by her adultery. This is done by describing one's sexual activities very exactly in a series of letters to the male church authorities. Believers must submit to this humiliating rule in order to avoid spending eternity with their ex-husbands, because they must be able to enter the temple to obtain a cancellation of sealing, required if a woman wishes to remarry in the temple. Women can be celestially married to only one man at a time. Men are not required to undergo any of this to get their temple recommends back, and they, of course, have no need to cancel the celestial marriage to one woman in order to marry a second" since men can have multiple eternal wives.

"Late LDS apostle Bruce R. McConkie wrote that the most important thing a woman can do is 'to marry the right person, in the right place, by the right authority.' It had been repeatedly impressed on me that if I failed to marry a faithful Mormon man in a Mormon temple, I would be denied access to the highest level of Mormon heaven . . . The temple marriage is so important that a longing for romance on earth should not be allowed to interfere with it.

"Girls and boys are told that a good and proper Mormon home is a patriarchal one. A handbook written for 14-year-old boys states that, *The patriarchal order is of divine origin and will continue throughout time and eternity.* Husbands conduct family prayers, bless wives and children, and generally control the household. The Mormon belief is that Eve's roles of help-mate and child-bearer set the pattern for her daughters.

"*Girls are told that God wants them at home, and boys are never taught to clean up after themselves, since when their mothers stop doing it for them, their wives will take over the job. These ideas have not changed at all since the 19th Century.*"

Like many religions, Mormons believe the female bears the guilt and responsibility for sexual wrongdoing – if a girl allows a boy or man to touch her, she will be damaged goods and no male will respect her, even though *he's* doing the molesting.

The strict chastity demanded of Mormon women conflicts with the mandate that women should please males in their lives. What does a girl or woman do when the boy or man she is with, who is inspired by God, wants to have sex?

LDS Temple Rituals

In 1990, the Mormon church implemented a dramatically revised temple ceremony. These rituals had been in the LDS temple ceremony for 160 years. Some key changes were:

- The creation and restoration story acted out in the temple had included a Protestant minister being paid by Satan to preach false doctrine. This was eliminated.
- The church also eliminated all penalties and gestures such as slashing the throat, cutting open the chest and disembowelment as punishment for telling temple secrets.
- The new ceremony modified the woman's promise to be obedient to her husband "as long as he follows God."
- The intimate position of the "veil between heaven and Earth" that temple worshipers, both men and women, had to place between them was foot-to-foot, knee-to-knee, breast-to-breast, hand-on-shoulder, and mouth-to-ear. This was eliminated.
- The chant *"Pay Lay Ale,"* meaning *"Oh God, hear the words of my mouth,"* was eliminated.

Critics say the changes made in 1990 were the result of an article in *Dialogue: A Journal of Mormon Thought* published in 1987 that revealed the most questionable temple rituals. The church conducted a survey of members in 1988, asking their opinions about the "endowment" ceremony. A significant number of members indicated various parts of the ceremony offended them. In particular, many converts with a Christian background balked at the minister being bribed by the devil and expressed discomfort with the bloody oaths.

The *Dialogue* article by John Buerger reads in part: "There were strong indications that Joseph Smith drew on Masonic temple rites in shaping the Mormon temple endowment, specifically borrowing the tokens, signs and penalties. The number of LDS temples has increased dramatically. But rates of temple work have remained constant over 15 years. Members of my own stake made 2,671 visits to the Oakland Temple in 1985, versus 3,340 visits in 1984, a 20% drop. The feelings contemporary Saints have for the temple certainly merit a careful quantitative analysis by professional social scientists. I have heard a number of themes from people who feel discomfort in one degree or another with elements of the temple ceremony.

"Probably in no other setting except college organizations, with their associations of youthfulness and immaturity, do most Mormons encounter secret ceremonies with code handshakes, clothing with particular significance, and implied violence of the penalties. Various individuals have commented on their difficulty in seeing these elements as religious or inspirational, originating from a Father for his children."

Most Mormons don't know what happens in the temple until they attend an "endowment" ceremony, usually at 19 years of age for males preparing for their missions and at whatever age females get married in the temple and have their first endowment.

Consider one LDS woman's description of that experience: "A lot of things bothered me about the ceremony, starting with where they asked if anyone in the room was not ready to agree to the promises they would be giving. That person was to raise their hand and they would be escorted out of the room. I wondered then why they would ask that when I didn't even know what I was going to promise!

"I felt very uneasy about that until I looked over at my mom and sisters. They were all smiling so I felt reassured. The film (enactment of the creation and restoration) turned me off right away. There's Adam and Eve. She is standing in the background the whole time while all the action is going on. No one talks to her or even looks her way! Then came all the handshakes and signs. I felt very weird about the words and the actions that accompanied them. I was seriously beginning to wonder what I had gotten myself into. Once I passed into the celestial room, we could all talk freely about the ceremony. The most common comment I got was, 'It's not what you would expect is it?' Damn straight it wasn't! *How could a person go through life in an organization and not even know how bizarre it was at the very heart of he thing?*"

It's All About Money

Being a Mormon is expensive. Members are expected to give 10% of their salary to the church. In fact, church members must pay a full tithe in order to receive a temple recommend which they must renew yearly.

TIME magazine published *"Mormons Inc."* in August 1997, reporting on the LDS church's vast wealth: "The Mormon church's current assets total a minimum of $30 billion. If the church were a corporation, its $5.9 billion in annual gross income would place it midway through the Fortune 500, a little below *Union Carbide* and the *Paine Webber Group* but bigger than *Nike* and *The Gap*. Most churches take in donations. Very few, however, impose a compulsory 10% income tax on their members. Last year $5.2 billion in tithes flowed into Salt Lake City. By contrast, the Evangelical Lutheran Church with comparable membership receives $1.7 billion a year in contributions."

A majority of the Mormon church's highest leaders (the general authorities and 12 apostles) make more than two to three times the average yearly salary of $38,884 earned by most heads of Utah households.

A *Deseret News* article published April 22, 1989, stated: "Advocates for Utah's poor are saying the state must admit it has a problem and then plan a strategy to deal with not only those on the welfare rolls but *the working poor that comprise a burgeoning economic class in Utah*. Steve Johnson of Utahns Against Hunger said, 'We always hear about the per capita, and they say it's our large families, but statistics show the individual Utah wage earner pulls in 10% to 15% less than the national average. We are a poor state.'"

Utah is a poor state where wealthy business owners, many of them active Mormons, don't pay a living wage and discourage (if not strong arm) employees from joining any union. Employers call Utah a "right to work" state. In actuality, this policy is a "right to fire" without giving cause or notice. This opens the door for racial, ethnic, age, gender and religious discrimination just like the "olden days," just like it was in other states a long, long time ago.

Some call these practices backward. I call them ancient, controlling and discriminatory. Without a union, Utah employers treat employees anyway they wish and get away with it. The rest of the nation is beyond this. Utah is stuck in it. In fact, the state economy depends on it. This way the powers-that-be can keep the population poor and under their thumb.

Chapter 5

Utah's Revealing Statistics

Is it merely a coincidence the most famous Mormons in the nation, Donny and Marie Osmond, have psychological disorders that can be traced to childhood trauma? Donny revealed to the world he has suffered from panic disorder that nearly ruined his career. Marie told television viewers that she was sexually abused while touring as a young singer. She recently sought treatment for severe depression after the birth of her last child.

This is certainly not their fault. Both Osmonds, now in their 40s, spent a lifetime pressured to be perfect. I believe their personal challenges are the result of being raised in a religion that ignores the needs of children and fosters mental illness.

Marie Osmond talked with *Entertainment Tonight* as she prepared to publish her book, *"Behind the Smile: My Journey Out of Postpartum Depression,"* concerning her lifelong battle with depression and her recent postpartum illness. "During my childhood and teen years, I was abused,' she said. "It ranged from invasions of privacy to having my personal property stolen, and, most damaging, being abused sexually."

Marie said her abuser threatened her. "I was terrified about my personal safety and that of my family," she said. "Although instinctively I knew the abuse was wrong, I pushed it down. I always knew it was there in some part of me. I struggled with my self-esteem every day."

An article by Dianna Ippolito in *Ability* magazine quotes Osmond about the day she left her children: "I basically gave the baby to the babysitter, gave her the credit card, got in my car and just really felt that my kids would be better off if they did not have a mother. I just left, never thinking I would come back, not really knowing where I was going or what I was doing."

She later sought therapy to heal the wounds of child sexual abuse: "I went to a psychologist and went through my problems and came out on the other end incredibly healthy. Things in my past that I really thought were over and done with were still elements of the puzzle that weren't pieced together.

"I would talk about sexual abuse and what it did to me, I felt like I couldn't write truthfully about postpartum depression without mentioning how (the molestation) skewed my thinking. I lost boundaries as a child that I didn't even realize it and it wasn't talked about back then. You know, it was something you just buried and dealt with, and moved forward. What could you do about it? . . . I became a bonafide workaholic. I can see now how it skewed my thinking. So, when I could no longer control these buried issues, I went crazy. I was so, so depressed. I could not find any joy. Nothing."

A few years ago, Donny Osmond was diagnosed with social anxiety disorder, a condition that causes an irrational fear of social or performance situations. He went through terrifying panic attacks. Donny described these attacks to Harold Dow on the television news program *48 Hours*.

"There are times I remember before I walked on stage where if I had the choice of walking on stage or dying, I would have chosen death," Donny said. He believes his problem has its origins in his childhood stardom. He started feeling anxious when he was about 11. "Ever since I started in the business, I knew at least somebody in that audience is looking at me all the time," he said. "So, I've got to be perfect."

Like many child celebrities, Donny had trouble making it as an adult star. When he was a hit in the musical *Joseph and the Amazing Technicolor Dreamcoat,* he felt even more stress:

104

"Now the pressure was even greater to be perfect," he said. "I thought I was actually going crazy in my mind. I remember shaking in bed, and I just, I couldn't get out of bed. Something was wrong, and my wife took me to the hospital.

"The problem I had, I didn't even know there was a name for it," he said. "The last thing I wanted to do was see a shrink, that would've ended up in the tabloids as *Donny Osmond is crazy.*"

He said he is doing better: "You know it's something that never leaves you. It has to do with a Type A personality, a perfectionist, those who really want to strive to achieve something a little bit greater, a bit higher and you're constantly kind of knocking yourself down if you make a mistake."

Marie said she, too, felt pressure to be perfect, and as a result poured herself into her career: "I found for me that my safe place was work. I could control my environment. I became very fastidious and detailed, and wanted things a certain way. Lots of times, when we feel out of control in certain areas, we find ways to control ourselves in other areas."

From The Mouths of Babes

Another well-known Mormon, Steve Benson, who won the 1993 Pulitzer Prize in editorial cartooning, denounced his membership in the LDS church after publicly revealing that his grandfather Ezra Taft Benson, the then president of the church, became incapacitated shortly after taking office in 1985.

The elder Benson was not leading the church yet Mormon authorities went to great lengths to perpetuate the illusion that their prophet still was functional, the younger Benson said. Steve Benson talked with *Associated Press* reporter Vern Anderson about the coverup on July 10, 1993. The final straw to break his silence was a comment his own son made one Sunday morning: "Why do they call grandpa a prophet when he can't do anything?"

"His own great-grandchildren could see it," Benson said. "Anyone could see it. It was a dirty family secret."

Soon after Benson talked with the media, the *Salt Lake Tribune* reported that the corporation which manages the LDS church transferred power to make corporate decisions from Ezra Taft Benson to his two counselors as early as 1989.

In November 1993, Steve Benson and his wife submitted their resignations from the LDS church.

Benson said: "I will not allow myself to be abused in this kind of dysfunctional system, where they try to manipulate me, control me, silence me, try to deny my right to speak out. Because if we don't have the individual right to speak out, what are we?"

Benson gave even more detailed reasons for leaving the church in an article he wrote May 1994 for the *Arizona Republic*, where he worked as a cartoonist. Again, Benson cited comments from his children that helped lead him to a dramatic change in his perception of his lifelong religion.

"Our oldest son seemed to understand the situation well. Months before we left the church, he made this unprompted observation: *Dad, I'll tell you why there's religion in the world – to control people by scaring them into believing that if they don't obey, they're going to hell,*" Benson wrote. His teenage daughter also let her misgivings about the church be known, especially concerning the treatment of women disrespected by LDS patriarchal authority.

"One day, she stood up in her Mormon-youth religion class and boldly told the teacher that just as the denial of the Mormon priesthood to black men had been racist, so the denial of the Mormon priesthood to women was sexist," Benson said.

Benson's wife, Mary Ann, experienced Mormon sexism first hand. "We became concerned with efforts by the Mormon patriarchy to stifle and control women," he said. Mary Ann was chastised by a Mormon male leader, who refused to deal directly with her but instead relayed his criticism through her husband. The leader said it was inappropriate for Mary Ann, in youth Sunday school class, to praise the courage of the female followers of Jesus, who remained at his side even through his death, while contrasting it to the actions of his male disciples, who fled for their lives. 'We wouldn't want the young men to think their priesthood leaders were less than loyal,' the church leader said."

Mary Ann Benson was especially concerned with how LDS leaders mishandled reports of child sexual abuse. *Priesthood authorities showed alarming ignorance and prejudice when it came to denying the severity of sexual abuse in the church and its impact on victims.* "Mary Ann was appalled at a patriarchal system that *protected pedophiles and minimized the pain suffered by victims of sexual abuse.* She was dismayed by a senior apostle's callous trivialization of the pain felt by abused women as *'comparable in the eternal scheme of things to a very, very bad experience in the second semester of the first grade.'"*

106

Who Is Responsible?

An official letter from Mormon officials *specifically about sexual abuse*, showed the church's lack of knowledge and compassion concerning adults molested as children. Church authorities advised priesthood leaders that an adult, adolescent or "mature person" who consents to sex with an aggressor (or abuser), must *"share responsibility for the act."*

This letter went out to LDS general authorities, regional representatives and other priesthood leaders Feb. 7, 1985: "Of course, a mature person who willingly consents to sexual relations must share responsibility for the acts even though the other participant was the aggressor. Persons who consciously invite sexual advances also have a share of responsibility for the behavior that follows. But persons who are truly forced into sexual relations are victims and are not guilty of any sexual sin."

When children or adolescents are abused repeatedly by adults, they often do not have the psychological or physical freedom to resist even when they become adults themselves, *(see case histories of Janet on page 37, and Deon on page 44.)* These people have been conditioned and programmed all their lives to be victims. They'll continue to act as the child victim especially if they have not received appropriate therapy to break the cycle, confront their abusers and take back their power.

President of the Quorum of the Twelve Apostles, Thomas S. Monson, has said: "Let the offender be brought to justice, to accountability, for his actions and receive professional treatment to curtail such wicked and devilish conduct. *When you and I know of such conduct and fail to take action to eradicate it, we become part of the problem. We share part of the guilt. We experience part of the punishment." (Ensign,* Nov. 1991, p. 69.)

This is what Monson said but the church as a whole and priesthood holders individually act just the opposite.

The Mormon church, in fact, has legally said priesthood leaders are not required nor duty-bound to act in the victim's interest when they hear reports of sexual abuse, *(see Franco case on page 16, and Scott case on page 17.)* The priesthood holders who hear of these atrocities are "part of the problem," they do "share the guilt," and they should "experience the punishment." Let Monson and fellow priesthood leaders practice what he self-righteously preaches.

Women & Children

Some 34% of Utah women report severe emotional abuse at home, according to the *Domestic Violence Incidence and Prevalence Study* conducted by Dan Jones & Associates in 1997. The study was used by Utah Attorney General Jan Graham when she published *SAFE 2000: Ending Abuse and Violence in Utah Families, How to Get from Here to There.*

"Women are also victimized through isolation, intimidation, economic threats, or threats to children," Graham's report said. "These forms of abuse are intended to control the victim, and are usually precursors to physical abuse."

About 40,000 women and 160,000 children in Utah suffer abuse at the hands of the adult males in their lives, the report said: "That means in an average public school classroom of 35 students, about 8 of them live in homes with violence or abuse. Sadly, 50% of these children are also being physically abused by the batterer." Experts in Utah estimate that more than 50% of women and children who visit emergency rooms do so for injuries inflicted intentionally at home.

Graham specifically addresses the roles that religion and churches must play in protecting women and children from abuse. "Many families dealing with abuse and violence have active affiliations with their church. Some 21% of women said they would turn to clergy first for help. Most clergy are at a loss as to what to do, and advice can often be devastating like, 'Go home and try harder.' Telling a victim that 'the most important thing is to keep the family together,' means a victim and her children are condemned to bear the brunt of abusive conduct," the report said.

Many women stated that clergy tend to minimize the problem or feel uncomfortable discussing it and want to "brush it aside." One woman said her husband abused her because she didn't keep the house clean enough, and her religious advisor encouraged her to keep the house cleaner.

The SAFE 2000 report concluded: "Church leadership is moral leadership, but what could be more immoral than abuse and violence toward a family member, toward a child? Silence and discomfort from religious leaders suggest that abuse and violence at home may not be immoral, or that it may be a 'private family matter,' which means that it should remain a family secret.

108

"It is time to change those perceptions by asking what a church can do to help families struggling with family violence: What specific training does a church provide to its clergy about domestic abuse? Do churches have support groups for their members? Do members of the clergy know where to refer women for professional help in escaping abuse? These must be in place to help victims of abuse move forward."

Sobering Utah Statistics

Utah statistics mirror deplorable national reports that show at least half of the women who reported being raped in 1992 were juveniles under 18 years old, and 16% were children younger than 12, according to a Department of Justice study.

Another report in 1991 showed that 96% of the female rape victims younger than 12 years old knew their attackers, and 20% were victimized by their fathers. Some 94% of state prisoners confined for child rape said their victims were family members, acquaintances or friends.

According to a Utah task force study entitled *When the Victim is a Child: Issues for Judges and Prosecutors*, child sexual abuse is perpetuated against about one-fourth of all female children. Much of this abuse is never reported. In Utah, *less than half of the cases* reported to Child Protective Services are substantiated due to lack of hard evidence and "adequate" disclosure from victims. *Only 2% of the cases where child sexual abuse is reported in Utah result in conviction.* Of 56 adult perpetrators studied for the report and referred to law enforcement for formal investigation, only 24 – *less than half* – were charged. Only five of those served time.

Charges are rarely filed against perpetrators whose cases have already been verified by Child Protective Services and police investigators. "The fact that nearly two-thirds of the substantiated cases referred to law enforcement were not prosecuted may be a cause for concern," the report states. 'Questions that should be addressed include: Can more of the cases be successfully prosecuted? To what extent are other actions taken to address the problem of offenders remaining free? What is being done to protect children in these cases?"

Prosecutors got convictions on 19 of the 20 molesters and rapists charged. *Only five of the 19 convicted criminals were sentenced to serve any time.* Seventeen defendants pled guilty, two were found guilty in trials, and one was acquitted. The expectation based on the minimum mandatory sentence law is all or most of the perpetrators would go to prison for 10 years. However, 14 of 19 convicted offenders got probation. Typically, this occurred as the result of plea bargains to lesser offenses.

The task force study answered few questions and raised many: "The fact that most convicted child sex abusers are not sentenced to prison and are not receiving minimum mandatory terms raises many questions. Does the minimum mandatory term encourage plea bargains? To what extent do the offenders who are granted probation recidivate? How effective are treatment programs inside and outside prison?

Utah Victim Characteristics

Victims of sexual abuse in Utah in 1988 were typically female (75%). Nearly half (47%) of the victims were between the ages of 6 and 11. Thirty percent were 12 years old and older, and 24% were 5 years old and under. Of the reported victims of sexual abuse, 22% previously had been victims.

Utah Offender Characteristics

In 61% of Utah cases studied, the perpetrator was related to the victim, 15% fathers, 14% siblings, 9% stepfathers, 9% uncles and the remaining were other relatives. Some 42% of perpetrators were 19 years old or younger. The next largest category were predators in their 30s (22%), followed by those in their 20s (16%).

Crisis Can't Be Ignored

When LDS church officials claim that Mormons don't have any more instances of child sexual abuse than the regular population, they are blatantly ignoring and denying the growing number of criminal cases and lawsuits that prove they do. The abuse in Utah is even more pronounced than recently publicized problems in the Catholic church chiefly because 1) more male members of the Mormon church act as clergy, 2) if they abuse children at church, they also likely abuse them at home, and 3) the behavior is innate to and generational in dysfunctional Mormon families. Thus, the opportunity and numbers are greater.

110

What is going on inside the heads of men who think they can rape and molest their own babies and others' offspring, live as racist, sexist and elitist patriarchs all of their earthly lives, then die and become Gods? What is wrong with this picture? That's not ignorance, that's culturally ingrained mental illness.

Consider these cases:

• During the mid-1980s, information emerged about a child sexual abuse and pornography ring run by two counselors in a Bountiful LDS bishopric. Eight children told their parents, police investigators and therapists how they were sexually abused by ward members. Only one person, Brett Bullock, was prosecuted. He is serving time in prison.

• In 1994, George P. Lee, a general authority and member of the First Quorum of the Seventy since 1975, admitted to sexually molesting a 12-year-old neighbor girl. Lee, 51, pleaded guilty to attempted sexual abuse of a child, a third-degree felony. The victim said Lee fondled her breasts, buttocks and genitals for three years, beginning in 1986 when she was 9 years old. Lee was excommunicated from the church in 1989.

• In 1996, Idaho senator Rex Furness spent two months in jail for sexually battering his teenage granddaughter. The charge against him forced him to resign from the senate. He was active in the Mormon church, holding various titles, including bishop until he confessed his acts and surrendered his temple recommend.

• In 1997, Lloyd Gerald Pond, 51, was charged with two counts of forcible sodomy on a 14-year-old girl he met at a Mormon ward. Pond was employed by the LDS church's public-relations department and hosted a nationwide radio program that promoted Mormon values. Pond's radio work included warnings about the evils of child abuse and pornography.

• That same year, LDS attorney Michael Shean, a Mormon seminary teacher in California, was convicted of sexually abusing young boys. A civil suit against the LDS church alleges gross negligence on the part of priesthood leaders who knew Shean was a pedophile. When he was a counselor in the bishopric, he had been excommunicated for abusing two boys who disclosed the molestation when they were on their missions. Later Shean was re-baptized and allowed again to work with young people.

111

Everybody Knew But
Nobody Told Police

In March 2000, Jay Toombs, a 43-year old Benson man accused of fondling a boy three times in the early 1990s, faced another charge and growing evidence that LDS church leaders knew of the abuse but did not tell law enforcement authorities. Police officials were so aghast upon learning of widespread knowledge – but only one report – of abuse, that they considered bringing failure-to-report charges against a West Valley City counselor and two LDS bishops.

An article published in the *Salt Lake Tribune* gave details: "The mother says she spoke of Toombs' misbehavior with boys from 1991 through 1999 to a counselor, two LDS bishops and Toombs' family, including his brother, an LDS stake president. 'I was always told to be patient with Jay, he was a good man. That's what I was told again and again and again. I was even given priesthood blessings that I had been chosen to help him,' she says.

"The bishops were inclined each time to tell police, the woman says, but later told her they had checked with church officials and *learned they did not have to report Toombs as long as he was repentant* and getting professional help. Neither bishop called police. Bishop Robert Owens knew the Cache County Sheriff's Office investigated Toombs in 1989 and bishop Brent Bryner knew of abuse four years earlier and only informed law enforcment in 1997.

"Jerry Toombs, an LDS stake president and Jay Toombs' older brother, says it is not true that he had been warned for years about Jay Toombs' alleged abuse. Jerry Toombs was in the spotlight last year when he recommended a convicted child abuser, Shonn M. Ricks of Benson, for a mission after the 23-year-old had served a 14-month sentence at the Utah State Prison. The mission call was withdrawn after the victim's outraged father complained.

"Robb Parrish, chief child abuse counsel in the Utah Attorney General's Office, says the urge to have sex with children, pedophilia, is a deep-seated aberration. *'It doesn't just go away. They are not just in need of a little counseling. Pedophiles need intensive intervention, with the threat of prosecution held over their heads. The confessional situation to an LDS bishop is not enough.'*"

Stake President Fails
To Help Two Children

The church is being sued in West Virginia after an LDS stake president failed to intervene when a father confessed to sexually molesting his 8-year-old son and 5-year-old daughter. The abuse continued for five more years before the father's arrest after he videotaped himself abusing the children, according to a news article published in the *Salt Lake Tribune*, Oct. 17, 1999:

"In August 1996 in West Virginia, a mother and her daughter filed suit accusing the Mormon church of failing to intervene when it knew a male priesthood holder was sexually abusing his own daughter. U.S. District Judge Elizabeth Hallanan said $750 million lawsuit deals with a crucial constitutional issue and should be heard in federal court.

"The lawsuit alleges church leaders knew of the sexual abuse that the woman's ex-husband inflicted on her daughter but did nothing about it until his arrest in 1994. James Adams Jr was sentenced to up to 185 years in prison in February for molesting his daughter and her brother between 1989 and 1994. Years before his arrest, Adams feared exposure and confessed to New River Virginia stake president Blair Meldrum, who counseled Adams and believed he had repented and reformed. Meldrum did not report the abuse to state authorities – as required by law – nor did he talk to or arrange counseling for the children.

"Church attorneys said: 'President Meldrum took the father at his word, believing that he truly intended to forsake his past conduct and gain repentance in the eyes of God.' After 18 months, Meldrum decided Adams had 'sufficiently repented,' they said. The victim's lawyer argues Meldrum should have obeyed West Virginia's child abuse reporting law. With sufficient training or supervision, Meldrum would not have taken Adams 'at his word,' instead, the bishop would have known pedophiles – no matter how repentant – minimize their sexual abuse of children and do not stop without therapy."

Church Covers Up 30 Years
Of Abuse By LDS Physician

On September 12, 1996, *The Idaho Statesman* published an article stating that more than 100 women had reported a Mormon doctor sexually abused them and that the church tried to cover-up the incidents that took place in Rexburg, Idaho, the home to the Mormon-run Ricks College.

113

The newspaper reported: "Bonneville County officials are investigating a report that a Mormon church official tried to discourage a girl from testifying that Rexburg physician LaVar Withers sexually abused her. No charge has been filed, and the LDS official, bishop Dean Andrus, denies the allegation. Special Prosecutor Dan Hawkley said Andrus may have violated Idaho's anti-witness intimidation law which carries a maximum penalty of five years in prison.

"Withers began serving a *30-day sentence* in jail after he pleaded guilty to one count of battery for sexually abusing girls and women over a 30-year period from 1965 through 1995. At least two of the victims were 13 years old when he molested them. Many victims alleged that church officials ignored their pleas for help or *actually discouraged them from pursuing charges* against the doctor.

"Meanwhile, some of the women who accused Withers of molesting them filed a class-action lawsuit against him. For now, five women are listed as plaintiffs. The Rape Response and Crime Victim Center of Idaho Falls reported that *more than 117* women have said Withers abused them. Because the conviction covered three decades, women with allegations too old to prosecute under the statute of limitations were able to testify at Withers' sentencing hearing."

In these cases, the victims are abused twice, first by the molester or rapist, then again by a religious organization that chooses the criminal over the wounded. Why is this? Mormon clergy seem more concerned about whether or not the "sinner" repents, than whether or not the innocent women and children are protected. The pedophile knows what he is doing is wrong, he's already had his chance to reform. Once the abuse is reported, LDS priesthood holders need to care for those who are being abused and let God take care of the soul of the rapist.

114

Chapter 6

Protecting The Children

Always look intently at every person in your child's life and circle, most especially adult males since these make up the majority of pedophiles. However, don't overlook adolescents and females. Until they pass your inspection, everyone is suspect. Do not think you can spot a perpetrator from a distance because then you may miss the molester in your own home, next door or at church. Pedophiles live a double life. One face is the normal nice guy; the other side is devious, secretive, clever, manipulative and mentally ill. Consciously or subconsciously, the predator is always looking for unprotected children to victimize.

If you suspect your child has been sexually molested or raped, here are some actions you can take:

Believe your child. Don't deny the problem no matter how hard it might be to accept this happened to your child. Never assume the child is making things up.

Give your child immediate reassurance. Let her know the abuse was not her fault. Tell her you will keep the abuser away and he cannot hurt her anymore. Let her talk.

Control your emotions. Stay calm. Fear and anger are normal reactions, but they can frighten your child. Be sure you don't blame, punish or embarrass your child.

Get Information. Ask your child some questions about the incident but do not quiz him too intently. Get the facts you need to make a report to Child Protective Services and police.

Call Child Protective Services at 1-800-678-9366 and report the abuse. Make an appointment with a case worker to meet with your child. This is the first step in prosecution of the abuser and getting professional help for the victim. If substantiated by the CPS worker, the case will then go to a police investigator.

Get your child immediate medical attention. Especially if the disclosure of abuse comes when your child also is suffering physical trauma, pain or injury from the abuse. If there is noticeable injury or intense pain, take him to the Emergency Room. Let the doctor know your child was molested or raped. Make an appointment with the child's doctor to check for internal injuries and sexually transmitted diseases.

Protect your child from any flashbacks or issues with mistrust of those who are to protect and care for her. *Do not* take the child back to the place where the abuse occurred such as the church, daycare or relative's home. If the abuse occurred at home by a sibling or parent, separate the victim from the abuser. Either call police to arrest the abuser or leave with your child or children and go to a domestic violence safe house. If that's not possible go to a relative's or friend's home. The safe house is best because you will get the professional help there to break the cycle of domestic violence and child sexual abuse.

Leave The Abuser

So many of the victims I spoke with said they told their mothers about the molestation, rape or incest, and their mothers stayed with the abuser anyway. Get out! *If you stay and continue to sacrifice your child or children to a pedophile, you are an accomplice.* In a lot of homes where children are being sexually abused, the mother is also abused emotionally, psychologically, physically and sexually. If you cannot stand up for yourself, you have the responsibility to stand up for your children. Leave the house. Leave the abuser. Seek help from professionals to protect yourself and your children.

116

Leaving takes courage and smarts. Statistics show that battered women are at most risk for being killed when they leave. Do not let this frighten you. Be aware and take appropriate actions to ensure the safety of you and your children. If you discover or your child tells you of sexual abuse, remain calm. Do not confront the abuser right then because you do not want the situation to escalate. He will feel exposed and backed into a corner or he will use the opportunity to try to minimize the abuse and convince you to stay, continuing to feed your child to the predator. Your main goal now is getting out alive. Reassure your child that both of you will be safe. *Then once the abuser is out of the house, leave.*

Be willing to leave everything behind. Things are easily replaced. Children are not. Take only essentials, clothes and personal hygiene items. One bag. Make phone calls in private. Know where you are going. Then, go.

Empower Your Children

The best way to prevent your children from ever having to disclose a traumatic incident of sexual abuse is to set firm and consistent behavioral boundaries with your children from the time they are very young – giving them plenty of opportunity to make choices and decisions for themselves. In time, this will help them set internal boundaries.

Having the opportunity to meet many children and families while living in Utah, I must honestly say that while observing the parent/child dynamic here, I've realized there exists a lack of parental consistency, protection and social controls. I believe this is a direct result of socio/religious programming and conditioning of LDS women and their children. Even the smallest children seem to disrespect their mothers, hitting and biting them, and ignoring directives. From my observations, fathers in Utah are often absent from child rearing. The mothers seem more concerned about being nice and speaking sweetly to their children than insisting on discipline or self-control.

I've developed an empowerment and behavior modification program – called the *Specials Program* – that has worked well in helping children, especially those who have been victimized, to gain control over their environment, make decisions, build their self-esteem and feel safe.

The program works best with children 6 or younger since these are the most formative years. Parents with older children can modify the program to fit their needs.

When a child feels capable, he or she also feels safe. Giving the child responsibility appropriate to his age helps build self-esteem and self-power. Remember, setting limits that your child can count on will help him feel sure of his environment. Routines give the child structure and stability. He may protest and regress to whining, crying or wanting mom to take care of things. Do not give in. This will only give him the message that he is not capable of handling things himself. Stay firm to teach him that he has the power to control himself and to manage his day.

Encourage your child to be a "big kid." Do *not* use the words "good girl" or "good boy" as this places a moral judgment on your child's behavior. Instead remind her what big girls do in certain situations and let her know that you believe she can do that too. You have faith in her. You believe in her. Praise her when she makes appropriate choices.

Setting Boundaries

If your child asks you to do something he can do himself, don't do it. "I know you can do that by yourself. You're a big boy!" If he protests and starts to act out, you might say firmly, "I'm not your maid. You've got to get your coat yourself. " (Make sure the coat is accessible.) Showing your child that you, too, have boundaries and will not be run over by a child or another adult, will instill in your child that she should not take advantage of other people and that she, too, can set limits about how other people treat her. You're teaching her not to be a doormat.

If your child tries to get you off track by protesting, interrupting, whining or even wanting a hug, let him know that you will answer his question after he does what you have asked. Repeat the directive without addressing his need until he returns to the task at hand.

Deal promptly and firmly with zero tolerance behaviors. Whenever your child says, "No!" to a directive or request, stop and tell her, "You do not tell me No!" Explain to her that if an adult or another child does something that hurts her or that she does not like, she can and should tell them, "No!" But when mom gives her a directive or task, then she should do it.

118

Other zero tolerance behaviors include hitting, biting, purposely hurting herself or others, damaging property, and acting out with tantrums during mealtimes or outings.

Managing Meltdowns

Orient your child to the task at hand or the activity you would like him to do. "We are going to the store, what's the first thing we do when we get into the car?" Allow him to answer, buckle up our seatbelts! Letting him answer helps him to own the activity and take responsibility for "big boy" behavior. He's not doing it because you told him to but because he knows it's a good idea.

"When we get the store I need to get just two things and I expect you to be a big boy. I want you to stay by me. Don't ask for any treats because we aren't going for treats." Give him only two or three directives so he can remember them. "Now, how do big boys act in the store?" Let him mirror or repeat what you just said back to you. "Ok, are you ready, let's go!" If you give your child a directive or reprimand, ask her, "Do you understand what you need to do? Yes or no?" Do not continue until she gives you a response. Again, this allows her to take responsibility for her own behavior instead of simply begrudgingly following your rules.

Have some fun. Use exaggerated voice and actions, animation and humor to get your child to do something that he may be resistant to or might not want to do. For example, if he whines that he doesn't want to pick up his toys or put his books away, you whine too. "Oh I know it's so hard to pick up that little block, (you're trying but it's not budging). We gotta do it if we want to work on the computer, go to bed, eat dinner, play outside, etc."

Also make things she really must do into things she really wants to do. For example, "I don't know if you can get in that bathtub or play quietly here, or jump into bed and cuddle with dolly, or play (practice) the piano, or help mom make dinner or do the dishes – have you been a big girl today? Ok then, go ahead."

If after orientation and animation your child still protests, whines or begins to tantrum, firmly tell her if she cannot "calm herself" or "get herself together" she will lose a *special* she has earned, *(see program description that follows.)* Then, count. "I'm going to count to three. If you are not calm (or do not do as I ask) by the time I get to three, you will lose your special. If she does not calm down, take the special away.

If she doesn't have a special to lose, have her earn a special by showing you that she can be a big girl. "Show me how you can calm down and you can earn a special." Help her remember to sit, breathe, count to five slowly, close her eyes, etc. to gain control over a tantrum.

Remind your child if he loses a special that it's just how the program works – "It's your choice to lose the special or not, it's not up to mom, this is how the program works." Even empathize. "Oh, I know, I hate it when that happens, sometimes mom doesn't get to do what she wants to do if I don't do the things I'm supposed to do either. It's disappointing. I know how you feel."

Using timeout: If your child is extremely tired, is having a particular emotional upset or is hungry, uncomfortable, thirsty, etc. he may persist toward a tantrum. Then be very firm. Stand up over him and have him look you in the eye. "If you continue this nonsense you will get a timeout. You have until (decide a time) to get yourself together, calm and under control." If he does have a meltdown, an all out tantrum, put him in a safe room and close the door. "You can talk with me when you are finished." Shut the door and let him cry it out. Make sure he cannot hurt himself.

My Body Is My Own

Do not bathe nude with your child. She needs to know her body is her own private domain. Supervise bath time and be in the bathroom if she takes a shower. Give her a set time when she needs to get out of the tub. Set a timer or show her the hands or numbers on the clock so she can be responsible for finishing up her bath on time.

Mom and children do not run around the house nude. If your child does this, don't shame him. Just tell him to get dressed or to get his towel or robe. Say, for example, "I know it's fun to be naked, but you gotta cover up."

If she gets hurt or has an "ouwee" *ask* her permission to check it out especially if in private areas or under her clothes. "Can I look at your chest to see if you're alright?" Do not proceed until she's gives a clear, "Yes." Teach your child that no one has the right to touch her body without her permission. Also teach her to keep a courteous and wise distance from adults, especially strangers, even if they seem friendly and their parents know them.

120

Child molesters will befriend a mother to get to her children. Teach your child not to jump up on people's laps or give a bunch of kisses to someone she barely knows. A lot of parents think this behavior is cute. In this day and age, especially in Utah, such behavior puts your child at great risk.

To discourage your child from getting hurt just to get attention, if she does bonk herself and it is not serious (which the majority are not) just say, "Oh Kaboom! That was a good one! Or Ouweee, shake it off tough girl." Do not entertain the crying or run to her rescue. If she persists, use humor to distract her and get her to laugh: "Whoa, what a big one. Call an ambulance!"

Give your child plenty of love, hugs and positive attention throughout the day to avoid having him look for that by exaggerating hurt or sickness, or insisting on his own way.

Encourage your child to earn time (by getting a special) to practice martial arts, self-defense or play fighting and wrestling for at least 15 minutes each day. Have her choose it, don't force her to practice. Make it a privilege she must earn. Spar with her, reminding her she has to block or kick. Good punch! Mom should block too but let your child get a good one in once in a while. She must ask permission to practice. If she comes up and sucker punches you, she loses her "martial arts" special for that day.

The Specials Program

The specials program is a token economy by which your child earns small cut-out pyramids (or buttons or stickers) called "specials" that he can turn in or redeem for special activities during the day. On a poster board, glue pictures of activities that he enjoys such as having a treat, riding his scooter, watching a video, using the computer, practicing martial arts, reading a special book, going on an outing, talking on the phone or doing crafts.

How To Earn A Pyramid Or "Special": Your child can earn pyramids to do any of her special activities on her chart. She can earn one pyramid each, for 1) being a big girl, that means no whining, hanging on mom, no hitting, no tantrums; 2) doing her morning routine and night routine; 3) doing as mom asks. She can earn more than three specials by doing extra tasks during the day or as a reward for behaving extremely well. Just make sure you have enough time for her to redeem her specials. The best time is usually after school and work between mealtime and bedtime.

Routine gives your child structure, promotes a feeling of security, teaches self-discipline and encourages independence.

The Morning Routine: Remind him as you're getting his breakfast how big boys act at mealtime. For the morning routine, he will need to finish up his breakfast, clean up his station, take his plate to the sink, wash his hands, brush his teeth, then brush his hair or allow you to fix his hair, and get dressed on his own (make sure his clothes, socks, underwear and shoes are accessible.) You'll likely have to remind him of each step along the way, but not more than once.

The Nighttime Routine: If possible, have your child help you prepare dinner. If not, have her play on her own as you do. She should eat up her dinner, take her dishes to the sink, help do the dishes, then it's playtime, homework time or time to redeem her specials. After that, it's bath time. Make sure her towel and pajamas are accessible. Let her dry and dress herself for bed, brush her teeth, then play quietly or read until bedtime. If she has earned a bedtime story, read to her, then lights out at a designated time. Let her turn out the lights and jump into bed.

Redeeming Pyramids or "Specials": The child can turn in or redeem his pyramids during the day, most especially between the time you get dinner and go to bed. At home, just tape up pyramids that he earns onto a daily activity chart, a calendar or just a piece of paper. On outings, let him take his pyramids with him in a special wallet or pouch that fits in his pocket.

Also if she has her pyramids with her, you can use them as leverage to affect behavior. For example, if she begins to act out, tell her she will lose one of those pyramids if she doesn't act like a big girl. Also take some specials with you to reward her with when she accomplishes behaviors you have directed her to do on outings or behaves especially well.

On mealtimes: If she says she doesn't want something, she must taste it once before she can reject it. Remind her that she should eat what is prepared or go to bed hungry.

On bedtime: Nighttime can be difficult, especially for the tiny victims of child sexual abuse. Often times they are afraid of the dark or of being left alone. Your child might say he is scared. Talk about it briefly. Then empower him.

122

Give your child a special toy or stuffed animal to protect. "Can you help your bear go to sleep? Sing him one of your favorite songs." Keep a "fighting" stick near your child's bed. Build him up, letting him know he can "kick monster butt" and that you will keep watch from your room. Don't coddle at bedtime or your child will expect it and fail to gain the inner strength he needs to feel safe and capable on his own.

On helping: Decide if your child really needs your help when she asks for it or if she's just wanting you to do it for her. "What do you need me to do?" If it's something she can do by herself, simply say, "No, you can do that all by yourself. You're a big girl. Let's see how fast your can do it. Ready, set go!" or tell her, "You need to at least give it a try before I can help you with it."

The *Specials Program*, when used correctly, will build your child's self esteem and help her set internal behavioral boundaries for herself. She won't have to look to you to tell her what to do. She will quickly begin to feel more capable and in control of her emotions, actions and environment. She'll learn to make choices and reap the consequences, whether positive or negative.

The *Specials Program* also works with older children. Parents usually just call it allowance. Older kids earn money by doing particular tasks or chores, then redeem it when they get to go out or buy something because they've acted responsibly throughout the day or week.

The magic of using a token economy is that you can employ consequences immediately by giving or taking back specials as they are tied to appropriate and inappropriate behaviors. A child learns best through natural consequences, however, sometimes the lesson is lost when the consequence comes too late or doesn't show up at all. The *Specials Program* is not bribing your child any more than getting a paycheck is a bribe to go to work for an adult. Earning your way is a valuable habit to develop in life, the earlier the better. Teaching your children responsibility early on will help them grow into able and happy big people.

Check out these books to help you help your children:

- *On the Safe Side: Teach Your Child to Be Safe, Strong and Street-Smart,* by Paula Statman

- *When Your Child Has Been Molested: A Parent's Guide to Healing and Recovery,* by Joyce Case

- *Helping Your Child Recover from Sexual Abuse,* by Caren Adams with Jennifer Fay

- *The Right Touch: A Read-Aloud Book to Help Prevent Child Sexual Abuse,* by Sandy Kleven and Jody Bergsma

- *Parenting with Love and Logic: Teaching Children Responsibility,* by Foster W. Cline and Jim Fay

Chapter 7

Healing The Adults

They call themselves MACs – *Mormons Molested As Children* – victims of child sexual molestation, rape and incest who share a unique history and similar obstacles in their lives. Coming together to face those challenges will give them the strength and the hope they need to heal. MACs are dedicated to stopping the cycle – now! They don't want their children to suffer the same secrecy, shame, self-hate and dysfunction they have suffered.

Most Mormon victims of child sexual abuse, especially girls and women, are taught to be very accommodating. Be kind. Speak softly. Don't ask too many questions or share your opinions. Help everyone else before you help yourself. MACs do not accept that role. They are bold, brave and growing in power.

MACs are the ones who will stand up in the women's Relief Society group and ask: "Who of you were sexually molested as children? We are meeting in a support group at my house right after church, I expect you all to be there. We have work to do." Still some of them decide to leave the church to pursue an independent spirituality, a daring move since Mormonism is all many of them have ever known.

These women and men have the courage and survival skills that will help them make dramatic changes in their lives. Now, they are learning healthy behaviors and better ways to cope with the distinct trials of the legacy left to them.

Well-known in many Mormon circles is a historical novel entitled *The Giant Joshua*, published in 1941 and written by Maurine Whipple, a descendent of polygamist Utah pioneers. The fictionalized history is one of the first depictions of the polygamist lifestyle in early Utah.

Whipple tells of young Clorinda Agatha MacIntyre's loss of freedom and innocence as the teenage plural wife of Abijah MacIntyre or "Handsome Mac" as he was known to followers. The book is loosely based on the life experiences of Whipple's own grandmother, Cornelia Agatha McAllister, one of the wives of John T. McAllister – "Grandpa Mac" – who settled with his families in St. George, Utah, in the 1850s.

"Clory," a bright, adventurous and social girl, was in love but not with Handsome Mac. Nonetheless, Abijah MacIntyre, already near 50, took Clorinda as his third wife and raped the 17-year-old on a riverbank when they arrived in the red sands of the Dixie Mission after a long trek 300 miles south of the Salt Lake Valley. It was done. She was now his wife for eternity.

For a longtime, Mormon friends and some family members ostracized Whipple for her frank telling of a girl's disillusionment with her oppressive religion and stifling fate as a plural wife. For young Mormons of the time, reading and possessing *The Giant Joshua* was a gutsy act of rebellion.

Some church officials even banned the book because, in its honesty, it went against what they thought should be a more proper portrayal of early Mormonism. Now, Whipple's novel serves as an accurate and detailed account of traditions and folklore common to families who settled southern Utah.

So, it seems, MACs have a historical textbook sympathetic to their plight. The legacy left by "Handsome Mac" and his kind does not have to doom another entire generation of Mormons and Utah children. The new MACs, *Mormons Molested As Children*, can make sure of that by becoming a force for change. As they come together, reveal the secret and seek the help they need to become healthy adults and parents, their positive metamorphosis will improve the future of this state.

126

These many survivors are assets to Utah as long as they ban together, demand to be heard and require that church and state leaders defend Utah's children and take child molesters and rapists to task. If you are a MAC, ask around about support groups. If you can't find one, start your own. You can attend group therapy sessions for Adults Molested As Children (AMACs) to gain an understanding of how such groups function and how much they assist survivors in moving ahead with their lives. You can also find support groups by calling any nearby mental health facility.

Seek out the advice of a professional therapist or social worker who would be willing to participate in your MAC survivors' group. If you cannot find one, simply getting together to discuss your concerns, disclose memories, work toward healing and make plans for social change that will benefit all who participate.

Take the steps that Becky took *(see page 55)* toward mending her life, realizing that healing from child sexual abuse is an ongoing journey. You will gain power to deal with life in healthier ways than you've done so in the past.

A Difficult Change

I have noticed that many Mormons, no matter how disillusioned they are with their church, do not want to leave it. As long as it works for them, there is no need to leave. But even for those who want to break free, the change is difficult if not impossible, or so it seems to them. The structure of Mormonism is all they know. They need only learn that there is a wide spiritual world out there waiting beyond the walls of the Church of Jesus Christ of Latter-day Saints.

Some Mormons summarily ignore or reject facts about the LDS religion even those facts that reveal policies or practices that may actually hurt or demean them. I expect that many Mormons will ignore or reject the facts I present in this book. All their lives, they have been tied to and deeply invested in the church, both spiritually and socially. The heavily invested Mormon will actively avoid anything that might challenge their long held beliefs.

From a very young age, Mormons invest time, emotion and make decisions concerning their future, based on their church. Children attend weekly classes, learning of the LDS plan of salvation, missionary work, marriage, family and temple work.

They are told there is no other right or good way to live than the Mormon way. Young boys are given the priesthood at 12 years old and participate in rituals that add to their investment. Then comes the mission and marriage for "time and all eternity" in the temple. Every year of their lives, Mormons put a whole bunch of time, money and emotional energy into their church. Soon that bundle becomes huge, and the more heavily invested the person is in the church, the harder they will strive their entire life to protect that investment. And the harder it is to leave even when they decide their religion does not work for them anymore.

I pray only that the victims of child sexual abuse will be able to work within or apart from the Mormon church to find the peace and healing they need to live healthier and happier lives.

Some Helpful Resources

These books have helped many victims of child sexual abuse come to see themselves as the strong survivors they have always been:

- *Paperdolls: A True Story of Childhood Sexual Abuse in a Mormon Neighborhood,* by April Scott and Carol Scott

- *Reclaiming Our Days: Meditations For Incest Survivors,* by Helena See

- *Repressed Memories: A Journey To Recovery from Sexual Abuse,* by Renee Fredrickson, Ph.D.

- *The Courage To Heal Workbook: For Men and Women Survivors of Child Sexual Abuse,* by Laura Davis

- *The Right to Innocence: Healing the Trauma of Childhood Sexual Abuse,* by Beverly Engel

- *Ghosts in the Bedroom: A Guide for Partners of Incest Survivors,* by Ken Graber

Chapter 8

Exposing The Perpetrators

The first, easiest and best way to expose child molesters, rapists and pedophiles is to tell. Tell the secret. Shout it out! Point your finger at them and continue pointing until someone notices. Make a bunch of noise.

Pedophiles are cowards. Their activities take place behind closed doors under a blanket of secrecy. Pick up the heavy rug of silence and child molesters will scatter like the cockroaches, the vermin, they are. If you are fast enough and brave enough, you can bring a heavy boot right down on top of them. Just put your foot down. Drop it. Listen to them crunch and see how they cower under the weight of scrutiny. We owe it to Utah's children to expose and punish criminals who dedicate their sick lives to victimizing the innocent. So, open your mouth. Share your story. Stand up for other victims of child sexual abuse. Help them. Encourage them to take a stand. Open your mouth and shout.

The second best way to expose perpetrators is to make sure laws are in place that make a child rapist pay for his or her crimes. Swift and severe punishment can be a deterrent. Punishment also is a necessity to insure that victims receive the closure they need and the justice they deserve.

Demand that law enforcement comes down hard on those who do not abide by existing laws concerning child sexual abuse. Make sure everyone knows that it is against the law not to report child sexual abuse when you are made aware of it. Utah law requires a person with knowledge of child sexual abuse to report the crime, and provides a penalty of up to six months in jail and a $1,000 fine for those who do not. Clergy are exempt from the law *only* if their sole source of knowledge of the abuse comes from a perpetrator's own confession. If the clergy member learns of the abuse from any other source, such as a victim or concerned friend, he is required to report it.

According to Utah's law, "any person" who has reason to believe a child is being abused or neglected is required to report to authorities. Mandatory reporting laws arose in the 1970s as child welfare advocates challenged a traditional view that abuse was a private family or church matter.

Utah's law, while supported by those in law enforcement, has been repeatedly attacked by the LDS Church, according to an article published August 2000 in *The Salt Lake Tribune:* "David McConkie, an attorney who represents The Church of Jesus Christ of Latter-day Saints, called Utah's reporting law vague and ambiguous. But police argue Utah's law is clear. Marilyn Sandberg, executive director of the Utah Chapter of the Child Abuse Prevention Center, said many clergy want to believe abuse will somehow stop spontaneously – an erroneous conclusion.

"Law enforcement in Utah has given clergy simple advice to follow: Police and prosecutors, noting the secrecy that often surround child sexual abuse, contend clergy members and others can avoid trouble by reporting anything suspicious and allowing authorities to investigate. Yet Mormon clergy have repeatedly ignored the mandatory reporting law. Declaring himself innocent of wrongdoing, LDS bishop Bruce Christensen plans to challenge the constitutionality of a Utah law that sometimes forces clergy to inform on members of their own flock. Christensen is the third Mormon bishop charged this year with failing to report. Bishop David Maxwell allegedly failed to report the rape of a 16-year-old girl by a 15-year-old boy. Also this year, a Washington County LDS bishop Brent Atkinson, was charged with failing to report a suspected case of child sex abuse."

Victims Study Rejected

A study done in 1995 by Karen E. Gerdes and Martha N. Beck sought to find answers on how victims of child sexual abuse were being treated within the LDS church. However, when the results were revealed it was met with open hostility from the LDS Church, according to a news story published in the *Houston Chronicle* on May 10, 1999: "The sexual abuse study was denounced or worst of all, largely ignored by church officials who still dismiss it four years later. The study, which Mormon leaders condemned as flawed, found that more than two-thirds of the women interviewed said they had bad experiences when they turned to Mormon clergymen for comfort and counsel. For a church that in recent years has faced numerous lawsuits accusing it of harboring, or at least failing to stop, pedophiles in its midst, Gerdes said she believed she and her colleagues were providing some helpful insights.

"The researchers reported that, out of 71 Mormon women who had suffered childhood sexual abuse, 49 told of having 'negative interactions' with the bishops in whom they had confided. The women who reported the negative encounters described the bishops as 'judgmental' in some cases, 'unbelieving' in others and 'protective of the perpetrators' in still other cases. The research also found that 50 of the 71 victims felt guilt or frustration for being admonished by 'the highest church authorities or local leaders to forgive their perpetrators.'"

A professional psychologist and member of the LDS church, Arleen Cromwell, also sought to help the church with its sexual abuse problems. However, after a turn-around and recanting by the psychologist, many people questioned whether the Mormon church was engaging in a deliberate cover-up in order to protect itself from litigation: "In a sworn affidavit Cromwell signed in February 1996, the Salt Lake City therapist detailed what she called a pattern in which sexually abused children had been shunned or mishandled by bishops. Cromwell noted in the affidavit, given for a lawsuit in which she agreed to testify against the church, that families of the abuse victims often sought help from bishops, who failed to get them the professional treatment they needed. She said bishops often made 'little effort to ensure the safety of victims or failed to report abuses to appropriate state authorities.' In many cases, the bishop is ignorant of the needs of the victim, and does not act to ensure that the victim is not further abused," said Cromwell, who had been involved in treating abuse patients in about 300 cases in Utah.

131

The therapist went on to note that in March 1992, she 'became so concerned with the disturbing pattern I had seen emerging among the clergy of my own church' that she wrote a letter to her stake president. It seemed bishops had a distrust of therapists which made them reluctant to refer victims to therapy." Then Cromwell recanted.

An attorney for the victim in a lawsuit against the church said: "You have to wonder why a woman who is a credible psychologist with impeccable credentials would turn right around and say, 'Never mind. I didn't mean it.' You don't have to be a rocket scientist to realize somebody from the church got to her."

Just because a person has a title, doesn't make them righteous or competent. In every counseling job I have had, I've been highly scrutinized, as it should be. Mormon priesthood authorities should go through no less. If they counsel people, especially about serious life-changing issues like child sexual abuse, they need to be qualified, educated and act responsibly.

In addition to demanding that church officials follow the law on mandatory reporting, we must also look at changing the statute of limitations on reporting child sexual abuse and strengthening the existing mandatory minimum sentencing of 10 years for those convicted of child sexual abuse. Right now, few child molesters and rapists serve any time in prison or jail. Many of them avoid the mandatory minimum by pleading to lesser charges. Public pressure — that means *you* — can change the tide to protect victims instead of abusers.

Chapter 9

Passages Of Empowerment

Each and every time I hear the music . . . it is my choice
if and when I'll dance, or merely walk away.

In my own life, I have been empowered by the different people I've met and the cultures and traditions I've had the opportunity to experience through those associations. Growing up in a multi-ethnic neighborhood seemed normal to me. It was not uncommon to see children of various cultures, races and religions laughing and playing together.

As an adult, I was blessed to meet a Jewish couple, Sonia "Sophie" and Henry Billys, who hired me to do some maintenance work on their property and around their home. Sometimes, I would visit with them when they wanted company. Since my own mother was in Utah, Mrs. Billys became my adopted Mom. I named my daughter after Sonia because she is a powerful little lady who stands less than 5 feet but has a towering sense of self. Mrs. Billys is also a gifted artist. Her beautiful paintings are quite popular in respected circles.

There exists some ignorant myth that blacks and Jews don't get along. The truth is we have an unshakable bond due to similar backgrounds of oppression and atrocities against our peoples. We care for one another. I am living proof of that. They respect me, I respect them and, what's more, we genuinely like each other as individuals.

The Billys introduced me to several of their friends, including a kind widow named Mrs. Pitluck. One day on a break for lunch, she was dishing me up some more of her delicious homemade split pea soup when I noticed dark black-blue numbers tattooed on her forearm. It shocked me. I had to stare for a moment and try to come to grips with what this permanent stamp on her delicate skin must mean to her – this number took away her identity as a human being when she and her family were branded like cattle in a Nazi concentration camp.

I thought of the chains of slavery in my own racial history. Those chains stripped an entire race of people of their humanity. Mrs. Pitluck confided in me that her father, her brothers and her uncles all were murdered by racism. We held hands; we shared tears and each other's anguish that day, solidifying our historical connection and our tie as friends.

We talked about how her people suffered under the evil nightmare that was Hitler's Holocaust. I shared with her my own experience with bigotry and bias, how I worked for civil rights and fought against prejudice after I returned from serving my country in the military. We acknowledged how from this oppression emerged people of substance, courage and great strength of body, mind and soul. Our shared pain and power united us. I learned that a 76-year-old wealthy Jewish woman and a working-class black man in his 30s had more in common than not.

When a whole group of people are isolated and grow up seeing only one side of the multifaceted human race, their perceptions get skewed. In my opinion, the Mormon church does a disservice by encouraging a mostly white, homogenous, myopic and sheltered lifestyle for its members. This cloistered existence promotes a bunker-type, us-against-them mentality. If Mormons can't reach out to others to help them with a debilitating scourge like child sexual abuse, then the problem gets buried and festers until it explodes into the epidemic we see today.

134

I have faith there is a solution to this generational disease of child sexual abuse in the Church of Jesus Christ of Latter-day Saints. The change will not be easy. Admitting you have a problem is the first step. That is why I've written this book, to expose the crisis in all its horrible light. The responsibility to eradicate child sexual molestation, rape and incest in this state lies chiefly with the population it involves – the families of Utah and the members and leaders of the LDS church.

The world population must also be made aware of the dangers this poses for society and humanity as a whole. We must come together and put pressure on Utah political and religious leaders to protect children and punish perpetrators. No matter who you are or what religion you profess, *if you care about children*, speak out against this epidemic and tell a family member, a friend, tell everyone about Utah's *White Lies*. Give someone you care about the gift of knowledge, because knowledge is power. Children, born and unborn, need our collective power.

A Time To Heal

In my lifetime, I have found great strength in the written word and in my music. For all those victims who are hurting and need to heal, for all those who feel powerless and need to be empowered, I share some of my lyrics of songs that have gotten me through. By reading them, I hope you will hear the music in your heart and choose to . . . dance.

We're Here For You
This is a song for all of the children of the world
Be you troubled, sad, lonely, lost in this world
There's someone out here to help you
If you're on the streets,
in a mansion,
in the ghetto,
We're here for you
We've got love for you
Despite all temptations that come your way
Remember tomorrow will bring love your way
We're here for you

Changing

Everywhere I look these days, prophesies coming true
That's why it's wise to read the work, it tells you what to do
Woman against man, man against his son
Daughter against her mother, evil's on the run
'Cause my God is changing
Yes he's changing, I know he's changing
Changing the face of the world
    When I think of all the things that man can't explain
    It only makes it obvious that life's not a game
    He made a miracle over here
    A miracle over there
    Better look out sinners, my God is everywhere
    Yes he's changing, I know he's changing
    Changing the face of the world
Life seems unpredictable at times, but that don't bother me
'Cause I know that Jesus is always watching me
I know, I know, he's changing
Changing the face of the world

On The Winning Side

There was a time when I was a sinning man
Yes, I was blind
I couldn't see in front of me
I didn't care about no one but me
But as time went on
I began to see
What the Lord had in store for me
    I'm on the winning side
    This love I have I cannot hide
    There's a new road I'm on,
    I'm going on
    'Cause he made me strong
There was a time
When I didn't know the Lord
I didn't know that God is real
My God is real
I'm on the winning side
There's a new road I'm on
He made me strong

136

One More Day

Holy, Jesus your name
Let me call on you
I know that you'll to ease my pain
Power, you got power
Glory above
For you are the Father of love
Without love
Without your love
In my life
Without Jesus, I would die
      Giving me one more day
      Giving me
      You're giving me
      I'm so glad about it
      Giving me one more day
      Giving me
      I can't live without it
      Giving me one more day
      Giving me
      And I'm gonna live to love
I want to thank you, Lord
Giving me one more day
Giving me
Counting my blessings everyday
I know your giving me
Without love in my life
Without your love
Without Jesus
Don't you know, I would die
Giving me one

The Sacred Ones
by Kristi Glissmeyer

We are the silent ones
Broken children with eyes round as fruit
Cloistered in closets
Cowering in corners
Climbing ceilings
And we hide
We hide to survive

We are the scrappy ones
Know-it-alls with smiles keen as knives
Sleeping with strangers
Slashing our skin
Stalking streets
And we survive
We survive to heal

We are the scary ones
Hard women with lines stark as night
Screaming at dreams
Shouting the secret
Shunning death
And we heal
We heal to live

We are the sacred ones
Mended souls with eyes deep as water
Breathing bold each day
Letting go the grief
Seizing serenity
And we live
We Live

Sometimes I Forget

Sometimes I forget that I am not at home. I am not in a place where I have people who love and care for me, a place where there are people of my culture in all phases of local, state and federal government and strong religious establishments, a place where I am represented and feel safe. Sometimes I forget that I am in a place where the children are raped and molested at more than twice the rate of most states, where wounded children grow up to be broken adults who raise dysfunctional families, where mood- and mind-altering drugs – Prozac, Paxil, Xanax, Loritab – are taken as often as aspirins are in other places.

Sometimes I forget that the people I meet here are oriented to a different place and time, a place where I am not treated fairly, where people of color are stared at as if from another planet. Sometimes I forget, I smile and say hello to people I pass on the street as the majority of them look the other way, frown or don't speak at all. Sometimes I forget that I am not at home, but that I am in one of the most racist places I've ever been in my life.

Sometimes I just want to forget that this is the place where the people in power and those who follow them are so wrapped up in generations of their own unquestioned beliefs and mental illness that normal association is seen as abnormal. This is the place – Utah, where the most innocent and vulnerable, the very young and the very old, are abused, neglected and ignored. This is the place where people of a different color, culture, ethnicity, race and religion are seen as suspect and treated with disdain, while the real danger lurks in these tidy white-washed homes and within the walls of the churches found on almost every street corner.

--AEIII